Follow the Learner: The Role of a Leader in Creating a Lean Culture

by
Dr. Sami Bahri, DDS

Edited by Alexis Schroeder

Lean Enterprise Institute
Cambridge, MA USA

May 2009

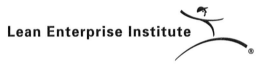

Lean Enterprise Institute

ISBN 978-1-934109-24-3
Design by Off-Piste Design
Printed in the USA
June 2012

Lean Enterprise Institute, Inc.
215 First Street, Cambridge, MA 02142 U.S.A.
Tel: 617-871-2900 • Fax: 617-871-2999 • lean.org

Table of Contents

From the Publisher

The purpose of *Follow the Learner* is to present a picture of how any organization can build a culture based on lean principles and tools. Why tell a story about a dental practice? First, everyone has been to the dentist. Every reader has a common frame of reference and therefore has experienced the processes and problems Dr. Bahri describes. Second, he happens to be one of the most dedicated and knowledgeable lean thinkers and practitioners in any field.

Bahri Dental Group is essentially a lean learning laboratory where Dr. Bahri is the "chief scientist" and this book is its lab report. It is designed to present a balanced picture of the technical lessons learned through 15+ years of creating a lean practice and the *leadership* lessons that support it.

Follow the Learner provides a glimpse into what it means to become a lean learning organization and a leadership model for continuously improving it. The Lean Enterprise Institute (LEI) hopes that people at all levels of lean experience in *any* type of organization will read this book to better understand the *universal* application of both lean methods and leadership practices. Bahri Dental Group is a microcosm of any service organization, and Dr. Bahri is a model for a leader as a learner and teacher.

Special thanks to each of the staff members at Bahri Dental Group for their inspiring stories and for their willingness to share them honestly; to the entire staff of LEI for providing their honest feedback and suggested improvements during the development of this publication; and to Off-Piste Design for bringing their impressive understanding of lean and dedication to good design to yet another LEI project.

Introduction

Walking into a dental practice in Jacksonville, FL one would hardly expect to find a learning laboratory for lean practices or a relentless lean pioneer. But that's exactly what I found when I first visited the offices of Dr. Sami Bahri in 2007. I had already heard about the "lean dentist" from lean thought leaders like Jim Womack and John Shook, and respected lean practitioners like Jerry Bussell from Medtronic. They all said the same thing, "You've got to see this guy ... He actually *gets it!*"

So what does it mean to "get it" when you're the leader of an organization, whether it's a dental practice with a dozen employees or a Fortune 500 company? Let's remember that the "it" we're talking about is *real* lean that strives to *consistently* deliver only value-creating services to the customer. The Lean Enterprise Institute (LEI) has chosen to share Sami Bahri's story because he has proven that he understands what a lean transformation requires of a leader:

- A deep understanding of how your customers define "value"and a willingness to build your organization around that definition

- Getting your hands dirty in the real work of your organization to understand where the value is flowing ... and where it's not

- Treating your organization as a system rather than a collection of disconnected operations

- A commitment to changing your own behavior while understanding what it takes to help others change

- A passion for learning—about your customer, your process and all of its problems, and about creative countermeasures based on constant experimentation

- An honest belief in the power of Plan-Do-Check-Act (PDCA) and a commitment to completing the improvement cycle *every* time

- Becoming the teacher who models lean thinking, participates in lean experiments, and learns/teaches by asking the right questions, rather than providing the right answers

- Humility to admit that knowledge is everywhere in the organization and that every improvement is temporary

Perhaps the most amazing part of this story is that Dr. Bahri is completely self-taught. Since opening his practice in Jacksonville in 1990, he has read virtually everything in the field of organizational improvement, from Deming's *Out of the Crisis*, to Womack and Jones' *Lean Thinking*, to Csíkszentmihályi's *Flow: The Psychology of Optimal Experience*. Even more importantly, he began experimenting with his staff to convert his new knowledge from theory to practice. So in the process of understanding what it means to be lean, he became the teacher for everyone on his staff (including fellow dentists), the scientific observer for his lean business experiments, and the leader of a lean enterprise.

Dr. Bahri has a profound understanding of the *essence* of lean. He got this understanding in much the same way as the original developers of the Toyota Production System. He pursued it because of an unshakable belief that there had to be a better way and through his own hands-on PDCA experiments.

It's been my great pleasure to get to know Sami well while bringing *Follow the Learner* to the market. The major challenge in the project has been to capture the deep understanding of lean that he has developed over his almost 30-year lean learning journey, while also preserving his gift for "keeping it simple." In the process, he's defined an equally "simple"—and very challenging—model of leadership. But these are the fundamentals, not the basics of lean leadership. If we've done our job, the book will help you to look at the fundamentals of your own lean implementation and the vital role that you must play in it as a leader within your organization.

We would also like to hear about both your successes and challenges and connect you with others in the lean community who might be tackling similar issues. Please contact us or the author by sending your comments and questions to: **info@lean.org**

Good luck!

Michael Brassard
President, Lean Learning Materials
Lean Enterprise Institute
May 2009

In Gratitude

My wife, Dr. Micheline Baz Bahri, DDS, told me one day: "*Well-timed acts of kindness seem very lean to me.*" The more I think about it, the more I find it to be relevant to the purpose of this book. Selflessly helping each other when needed, in the amount needed, is at the heart of just-in-time. After we have applied the technical aspects of lean, we have found that human relations come back constantly as the most important factor for the success of our lean transformation.

To my wife I say thank you—for bearing with me when I studied lean and when I prepared this book, and for taking such a good care of our family.

My love and thanks to the most precious Carol and Michelle, our two lovely daughters. Your experimentation at home, with "batch-and-queue" and "one-piece flow," have been very inspiring. No matter what business you select, I hope that the principles in this book will help you to run it efficiently. I hope that my lifelong work will contribute to making the world a better place for you.

Sami Bahri
May 2009

Part I: Creating a Lean Practice

In this first section, Dr. Sami Bahri describes the evolution of Bahri Dental Group's lean dental processes. What began in the 1980s with a personal commitment to reduce the long lead times before treatment, eventually led Dr. Bahri to "flow" the entire treatment system. He shares the "why" of lean, as well as the many experiments that he and his team undertook in order to learn and live a lean method of meeting the needs of every patient.

Because lean has its roots in manufacturing, some of the terms in this section may be unfamiliar to readers with service or healthcare backgrounds. At the end of this chapter (pp. 30–34) you'll find a chart of lean terms and their application in manufacturing and dentistry. This chart will also be helpful to readers in manufacturing who may want to see how familiar lean concepts and tools can be applied in nontraditional ways.

1980–2004 Searching for a Better Way

In the 30 years I have practiced dentistry I have witnessed the effect of long lead times on patients' health. In the old system, treatment was performed in multiple visits scheduled around the dental care providers' time. I saw patients postpone care and reschedule appointments until small cavities became large; until pain or discomfort forced them to come back for treatment. I saw patients who never get their entire mouths healthy again. Rather than lose time from work, they delayed treatment until more cavities were found when they came back for a cleaning, and the cycle repeated itself.

My quest for a better management system began on a trip to Paris in 1980, during which I read a few French and American books on dental management. While these books got me thinking about a few good improvements I could make within my office, I felt there was only so much I could learn from them. Something was missing.

1980

I wonder if other people have found a better way to do it?

This has been my guiding question ever since I opened my first dental practice. As soon as I had my first patient, improving the quality and efficiency of my service became a burning issue for me. The dental schools I attended in Beirut and Paris had not prepared me at all for the business side of dentistry; they had focused nearly exclusively on developing my clinical knowledge and skills. Some of my colleagues were kind enough to share their personal experiences at managing their dental offices with me, which was helpful, but unfortunately raised more questions in my mind than answers.

1984

In April 1984, I was appointed the first director of the newly created School of Dental Medicine at the government-run Lebanese University. Once more I found myself in a managerial position with no real management experience. Reading more books, talking to people with more experience than I had, and relying on my gut instincts worked well enough for a time, but I knew I was far from where I wanted to be as a manager.

1990

In 1990, I opened my new dental practice in Jacksonville, FL— Bahri Dental Group. For the third time, I found myself in the same uncomfortable position of starting a new project without a clear management approach.

I couldn't help but laugh at myself when on her second day, my front desk assistant came into my office and said, "Doctor, we have nothing at the front desk. We need a lot of things." I had no idea what "front desk" really meant, let alone what she needed to perform her job. She went to the store and bought our first round of front desk supplies. After she went home that night, I stayed at the office to look through what she bought so that I could better understand how she viewed her tasks at the front desk.

1993

By this time our practice was growing steadily. We had hired a few more employees, which helped us accommodate our increasing number of patients, but made management even more complex. In the midst of trying to keep up with our growing business and all the daily tasks that needed to be completed, I kept returning to the idea that there had to be a better way to do it all.

As I'd done since the 1980s, I continued reading about management in order to find that better way. I began learning about Total Quality Management (TQM) when a physician friend for whom I have great respect recommended that I look at the work of Dr. W. Edwards Deming. I studied Mary Walton's book, *The Deming Management Method,* and tried applying as many tools and principles of Statistical Process Control (SPC) as was practical. As always, I taught myself all of these tools first to prove that they actually worked.

1994

As I learned these new tools to improve the practice, I started training our staff to use them. I asked the staff to dedicate every Thursday to training. Many people were skeptical at first, but they seemed to like the idea of doing something different one day per week. Besides basic SPC tools, we would all learn other TQM tools like cause-and-effect (fishbone) diagrams by using them extensively to solve problems and make our daily work easier. More important than mastering the tools, we were learning how to think as a team about our daily work. I was learning how to present new ideas to my staff in such a way that they would not push back. We were all learning how to listen to each other and openly discuss problems together. When this happens anything is possible.

Around this time I discovered Masaaki Imai's book, *Kaizen*. It contained the tools of TQM, but also helped me understand the basic principles of the Toyota Production System (TPS). Looking back I see that it allowed for a smooth transition from TQM to TPS. I came out with a clear understanding that cross-training and employee suggestions were crucial for any business. This fit very well with Dr. Deming's teachings about breaking down barriers between departments and driving fear out of the workplace. From here we decided to start some serious cross-training efforts between hygienists, dental assistants, and our front desk staff.

1996–2004

In 1996, I came across an audio book that changed my life, *Lean Thinking* by Jim Womack and Dan Jones. I listened to this CD several times and then decided I wanted to go to the original referenced texts written by Toyota executives and insiders and read them firsthand, rather than accept another person's interpretation of them. I see now that I was following the Toyota principle "go and see for yourself"[1] before I knew anything about it.

1. Liker, Jeffrey, *The Toyota Way*. New York: McGraw-Hill, 2004. p. 223.

I started with *The Toyota Production System: Beyond Large-Scale Production* by Taiichi Ohno, the Toyota executive widely recognized as the "father of TPS," and *A Study of the Toyota Production System* by Shigeo Shingo, a consultant to Toyota known for developing key components of TPS. Then I started reading LEI's workbooks: *Learning to See, Creating Continuous Flow, Making Materials Flow, Creating Level Pull,* and *Seeing the Whole.* These books were by far the single most important source of information to me during this time. They helped me understand the practical aspects of lean management. It would have taken me many more years to apply lean to dentistry if not for these workbooks.

People often ask how it occurred to me to try implementing lean in my practice. What initially attracted me to lean was what I knew about its foundation in TPS. I knew about Toyota's track record: Toyota had grown steadily over the last 60 years to become the most successful automaker in today's market. This growth seemed very well controlled by its production system, which gave me the hope that by learning TPS and lean, I could exercise more control over the future of my business as well.

Truthfully, lean was one of several things we tried over the years in an effort to improve our practice. All I knew is that we needed to improve our operations and level of service dramatically. I saw that lean was about finding chronic problems and then eliminating their root causes to prevent future mistakes. As this became more natural, lean began interacting with everyday problems in a sort of dialogue that suddenly brought my business to life.

By 2004, lean had helped create solutions to all kinds of problems and dramatically changed the way we worked. Our early efforts were well received by patients, but one major problem stayed very visible and unsolved: patient wait times were still very lengthy.

We were constantly running behind schedule. No matter how hard we tried, we could not treat our patients at their scheduled appointment time. We tried many typical waiting room solutions. We placed television sets in the room and provided patients with a wide range of reading materials to make their waiting experience more tolerable. But we could find no real solution to the waiting problem, which made us feel helpless and frustrated.

I think the thing that stood out the most for me was the way Dr. Bahri was really open to change, even if it seemed completely against his logic. He's really open to new ideas. That's probably why lean works so well with his personality.

— Sarah Atkins
Patient Relations

2005 The Pursuit of One-Patient Flow

2005 was the most significant year in the life of our practice because this is when we started to create a new treatment system that would truly deliver one-patient flow. The frustrating scheduling problem that I've described triggered all of the changes in our system.

One day an incident caused us to look at our scheduling problem differently. A patient called about her daughter, who was studying law at Georgetown University and was coming home to Jacksonville for a week break. She asked if we could check and treat her teeth during her stay. We found that her daughter needed seven onlays and two composite fillings. Because she was short on time, we had to finish her entire treatment in one visit. It took us from 9:00 a.m. to 1:00 p.m., a four-hour visit!

I wondered: *Why couldn't we do this for all our patients? Aren't most of our patients short on time?* Most of them were either businesspeople or young mothers with children. This convinced me that we needed to take lean another step further. We were eliminating waste and implementing continuous improvement efforts, but did we really understand what these things were?

I asked my staff to think with me: *What is waste? What is improvement?* I went back to *Lean Thinking* to try to answer these questions. The book begins with a discussion of *muda* ("waste" in Japanese) and how we must eliminate it. I had a problem understanding this concept of waste elimination. When waste is defined as "any human activity which absorbs resources but creates no *value*,"[2] it can be confusing to the inexperienced student.

2. Womack, James and Daniel Jones. *Lean Thinking*. New York: Simon & Schuster, 1996. p.15.

Later in the book, Jim asks his daughter why she is folding her mom's newsletters in batches rather than one at a time. "Because it would not be efficient," she says. Reading this story was a revelation! I would have given Jim the same answer, but he wanted the reader to understand that there was a different way of doing things.

Later I learned it was what Toyota called *one-piece/continuous flow*. Real improvement at Bahri Dental Group only happened when we began directing our efforts toward this goal. What is one-piece flow and why did it make such a big difference? It is "producing and moving one item at a time (or a small and consistent batch of items) through a series of processing steps as continuously as possible, with each step making just what is requested by the next step."[3]

In manufacturing, this is very different from the traditional "batch-and-queue" approach in which you produce lots of the same part and it sits as inventory waiting to be used. One-piece flow has several major advantages: First, it forces you to always *add value* to your product (make it bigger/smaller, add a necessary component, etc.) rather than *waste* (waiting, transporting, etc.).

Second, problems can be identified and corrected quickly because the part is used right away, avoiding waste due to scrapping bad parts and delays in shipments. Finally, it allows you to change production plans quickly because you have little or no inventory to work through.

Why did this revelation have such a big impact on my practice? Strange as it may sound, I realized that a dental practice is not unlike a factory. For example, setups (the staging of the necessary tools and materials in preparation for any job) are almost as common and just

---

3. *Lean Lexicon*. Cambridge, MA: Lean Enterprise Institute, 2008. p. 10.

as wasteful in a dental practice as they are in the average factory. Dentists often change instruments and materials when going from one procedure to the next—for example, from a filling to a root canal. In fact, conventional dental training told us to schedule patients by "batching" similar procedures so that we could avoid setups! I understand now that we were "batching and queuing" our patients based on what was easiest for our system, not on the needs of our patients.

From then on I decided that we needed to direct our energies toward trying to achieve what we called *one-patient flow*. This meant focusing on *providing our patients with the correct treatment they need, when they need it, in the right quantity that they need it, while eliminating anything that interrupts or delays this flow*. The whole treatment team (dentist, hygienist, and office staff) must work together to first understand what every patient *needs* medically and also what they *want* as customers paying for a service like any other. Then we can work to provide these things to them to the best of our ability.

Once I realized this, my job became much clearer: I had to work with my staff to design a system that would deliver (flow) quality treatment to patients every day. Just as importantly, I had to make sure that we surfaced and solved any problems that blocked this flow. According to Dr. Deming, as a leader I now owned the "system" and its constant improvement.

I would like to say that I had a well-designed master plan to reach one-patient flow, but I didn't. Instead, the story of our lean transformation felt much more like a long trek through a mountain range. Our learning journey was not a straight line. We started from base camp with a goal of achieving one-patient flow and, in as many cases as possible, completing all treatments in one visit. But as we set out to do this, we encountered one barrier after another. These barriers were like a series of mountain peaks. We needed to scale one peak before we could see the next one.

It has been my experience in implementing lean that, when you solve problems and overcome barriers, you can then see more clearly the next set of problems that must be solved—countermeasures that must be created. As we went through the many peaks and valleys during 2005, we all learned valuable lessons from every step along the way. The most valuable lesson for me was that everyone had to make the trek with me or I would be left standing alone at the top of one of those mountain peaks with a great view and no way to move forward.

So what did our trek toward one-patient flow look like? I'll try to present it the way we saw it—as a series of barriers and counter-measures—beginning with our decision to change setups. These descriptions won't include everything we tried, but rather focus on the experiments and learning that proved to be most important.

Barrier #1: Setups took up a large part of the appointment time. If a patient came to us for a simple filling and in the course of doing this procedure we discovered that the patient needed a crown on that same tooth or another, an assistant had to change setups to prepare for the crown procedure. The change often took so long to complete that we (and the patient) were discouraged from performing the crown during that same appointment.

Countermeasure: Simplify cassettes and storage of supplies.
Setups involve what we call cassettes, sterilizable metal trays holding up to 30 instruments. Each procedure we do requires its own cassette. I asked the other dentists to try to notice how often each instrument in the cassettes were actually used.

After a few months, we realized that about 90% of the procedures only called for 10 or 11 instruments. We decided to change the cassettes to include just those instruments. The additional ones were stored in nearby sterile pouches in each of the patient rooms to be used when needed. Soon enough, our dental assistants were spending just a few minutes on setups for all dental procedures.

Setups also involve the materials used for dental treatment. We used to store materials in large bins called *tubs*. Each tub was dedicated to a specific process—one tub for fillings, one for crowns or root canals, and so forth.

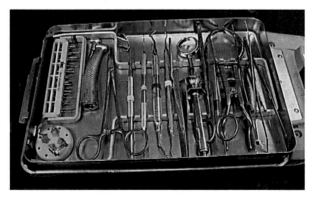
Reorganized instrument cassette

Simplified Supply Bin Storage

- *Right-sized* – small standard inventory, replenished daily
- *Visible* – clear plastic, eye-level
- *Comprehensive* – supplies required for 90% of all possible procedures
- *Accessible* – within reach, in every patient room

To eliminate the need for changing tubs when changing processes, we fashioned a new bin system; it kept all the materials nearby, ready to be used by the dental team. This reduction in instrument and material setups freed up a considerable amount of working time. The question now was how to spend it.

Barrier #2: Extra capacity.
When the instruments and supplies became available with little effort, treatments started to take less time. Eventually, we often found ourselves standing in the hallway of the treatment area, waiting for the next patient. I thought, *We need to schedule more patients to keep ourselves busy.*

Countermeasure: Have dentists perform all treatments in one visit.
I was about to ask the front desk assistants to add more patients to the schedule when I realized that a patient we had just dismissed needed more treatment and had made another appointment to come back for it. It occurred to me that our patients might be willing to undergo multiple different treatments in one visit, so I started asking them how they felt about the idea. The potential benefits were huge for patients, staff, and dentists. Consider the steps in a typical visit:

1. Check in the patient
2. Seat the patient
3. Numb the tooth and surrounding area
4. Prepare the tooth for treatment
5. Take X-rays
6. Treat the tooth or gums
7. Collect payment
8. Write a prescription, if necessary
9. Update the dental chart
10. Schedule the next appointment

Imagine a patient needing three office visits to complete a treatment plan. The same 10 steps are repeated for each visit, *but from the patient's perspective* only step six adds value. If the dentist and hygienist could complete all the value-adding work in one visit, the patient does the first five steps and the last three only once, instead of three separate times.

Most everyone responded positively, so we went on to finishing the whole treatment in the same appointment whenever possible. This would make the best use of our patients' time. We started doing all the fillings, onlays, and root canals, for example, in the same appointment when patients were able and willing to have us do so. Then I realized that if we truly wanted our patients to receive all the care they needed in one visit, cleanings and restorations should be done during the visit. But how could we offer both hygiene and dental treatments to patients within a reasonable time frame? There was no way we'd be able to do this as long as hygiene and dentistry were functionally separate, as they are in most dental practices. Our next barrier to one-patient flow was in sight.

Barrier #3: Hygiene and dentistry were functionally separate within the practice.
The treatment chairs in our practice were dedicated. Some were used exclusively by hygienists for hygiene treatments, and some exclusively by the dentist and assistant for general dentistry.

Countermeasure: Distribute procedures evenly throughout the schedule (leveling) to allow for combined dentistry and hygiene.
It just came to me: *The patient is coming to get whatever dental work completed that he or she needs. It doesn't matter where it's done. Why should we have specialized spaces when the patient has a variety of needs?*

At the time, the workload for cleaning (our most common procedure) varied greatly day-to-day. Some days the two office hygienists didn't have enough work to keep them busy; other days we had to have a third hygienist's help. On the busiest days the dedicated hygiene treatment chair was occupied every minute of the workday.

In December of 2005, I realized that if we wanted to create a single "treatment chair," we would have to restructure our existing schedule method, which was based on the number of hygienists and patient rooms—our office capacity. Each hygienist had a designated chair and time for cleaning—one hour. This approach severely limited our capacity and ignored the real, fluctuating demand for cleanings, which caused a very uneven workload. We desperately needed a more level and flexible schedule.

We learned that in lean you must first understand and evaluate your customer demand before scheduling your work, so we tried to forecast the following year's demand for cleanings. This would tell us how many cleanings we would need to complete during the course of a typical year to meet the needs of our patients. This was an ideal opportunity to use the very important lean measurement, *takt time*. In our practice we defined takt time as *the time required to complete an individual procedure to meet the total patient demand for that procedure during the course of a year*.

Let us assume for a moment that all our patients were willing to accommodate our schedule and allow their cleanings to be performed back-to-back during the entire year. Let us also assume that each patient entered the treatment room at the precise time of his or her appointment. The hygienist would have to finish a cleaning before the next patient arrives in order to have an empty chair for the new patient. The time from the start of a patient's cleaning to the arrival of the next patient is the required takt time for a cleaning.

We used the number of cleanings we had performed throughout the year to estimate our customer demand for cleanings. We divided the number of minutes we worked in 2005 (a total available work time of 104,160 minutes) by the number of performed cleanings (3,985 cleanings) to equal 26.13 minutes, which we rounded down to a takt time of 26 minutes. That means that, if a hygienist could perform every cleaning within 26 minutes, she would be able to complete all requested cleanings to meet the total yearly demand. But, was it possible to finish a cleaning within the required 26-minute takt time?

To answer that question, we determined our cycle time—how long it actually took to do a cleaning. When we studied the hygienists work, we discovered that a cleaning could be done in 21 minutes, which was five minutes less than takt time. This was after nonvalue-adding activities, such as walking to dentists' cubicles and cleaning up between patients, were eliminated. To eliminate some of these

> It's a total paradigm shift from what goes on in other dental offices. We've taken the approach that when the patient sits down in a chair they can receive dental education, their cleaning, and any treatment because we are set up in each room to treat everything. As dentists it gives us better control over what we are doing. From a patient's perception, it means fewer overall visits.
>
> — Dr. Anjali Lueck, DMD
> Associate Dentist

nonvalue-adding activities for the hygienists, we moved doctors and hygienists closer to one another to minimize walking distances, and we had dental assistants perform cleanups, collect payments, present treatment plans, and make additional appointments.

Using takt time and cycle time data, we could calculate the number of hygienists needed to meet the rate of demand for cleanings, instead of applying the traditional dental management formula of having one or two hygienists per dentist. In fact, the data showed us that only one hygienist was theoretically sufficient, if the load could be leveled all the time—not realistic given patient circumstances out of our control.

We were all impressed with the data so we decided to divide the load among two hygienists, not replacing a third hygienist who was leaving the practice for personal reasons. We found that we could meet the demand by performing 12 cleanings a day, split between our two hygienists. We went from three full-time hygienists before our takt time study, to two hygienists working half of the time after it.

What did they do during the four hours remaining in the day? Our new system provided for more than a 100% growth, rather than the 10% we had planned for based on growth-rate trends from previous years. More importantly, with this new capacity and flexibility we were now able to accommodate new patients on short notice. It was not unusual to see patients leaving their treatment with their exams and cleanings finished, within two or three hours of their very first call to our office.

The flexibility of our staff and time allowed us to meet the growing volume of patients without having to add staff. We had no more dedicated treatment rooms; all rooms were common to dentists and hygienists and were now called *patient rooms*.

All of these changes were great improvements, but there was a new barrier to overcome. Starting our *combined treatment* created major coordination problems because the daily schedule was no longer carved in stone. Patients were going into patient rooms for cleanings or dental work, or both, and the dentist and hygienists were now coming to them. But how would dentists and hygienists know where to go and when? After I was done treating one patient, how would I know where and when I was needed if changes had been made to the day's schedule or if a patient required additional treatment? If I was now going to be *pulled* into a patient's treatment, I would need a *pull signal*, but how could this be done?

Barrier #4: Lack of coordination between staff.
By now we were focused on flowing quality care to patients. The problem was that we didn't have a systematic method for changing direction once adjustments were made to the schedule.

Countermeasure: Create the flow manager position.
I wondered, *How did Toyota solve this problem?* They used the position of supervisor or team leader. We created a new position called the *patient care flow manager* to help maintain one-patient flow within the practice. We chose the title of flow manager to emphasize that it is this person's responsibility to make sure we are synchronizing our efforts around the needs of the patient, while also adjusting to

I used to deal with most of the large treatment plans, so I had my own office … That was the majority of my job over the years, being in an office, not out on the floor. After lean we eliminated the office. I have more patient and employee contact now. I make sure the providers are working, that the patients are being taken care of, that the flow is going. If there is a stop or a pause with the patient in the chair, I should be there to see what the problem is, see what can we do to continue the process with that patient …

— Candice Johnson
Patient Care Flow
Manager

inevitable changes that happen to our daily schedule. Their job is *not* to ensure that all employees are busy at *all* times (like running a machine at 100% capacity). Rather, they coordinate the movement of different staff so that a *patient's treatment is continuous* from the moment they walk in the door to the end of their visit. The flow manager guides everyone in the office, directing doctors, hygienists, and assistants toward their next move so that the patient's treatment never stops.

This shift of focus from *staff* productivity to *patient* productivity is by far the biggest difference between a traditional practice and a lean one. Staff have more joint decision-making power this way. Because doctors and hygienists are not used to being told where to go, our new system depends on their flexibility. But the benefits of flow managers are clear. Patients appreciate not having to wait and like the option of undergoing multiple treatments in one visit. The flow manager is always there to provide assistance and to see that the patient is taken care of at all times. In a ball game, it would be like keeping our eye on the ball rather than worrying about what other players—especially those not directly involved in the play—are doing.

Barrier #5: Flow manager has difficulty communicating clear and timely instructions to staff.

The flow manager knew how to direct staff members where they were most needed. However, people often clustered around her, competing for her attention. Because this caused delays, they started bypassing her and making their own decisions as to where to go next. This chaos forced us to immediately enhance communication between the flow manager and the rest of the team.

Countermeasure: Develop a visual system that communicates requests for service to all providers (service kanban).

When we discussed this problem in our morning meeting, we knew that *kanban* was the answer. That's how Toyota solves communication problems on its production line, by *telling the previous step in the process exactly when and how much they should produce of a particular part or product.* Ironically, I had promised my staff in 1997 that I would figure out how to use a kanban in dentistry!

Once again *real solutions* must start from *real needs*. The conditions for using a kanban were finally right because we knew something like it was necessary to make our new system work. We also knew that our solution had to fit our situation; we could not just copy it from another source. I suggested that we base the kanban on a cross-functional flowchart. The team members took the chart, adapted it to the needs of their jobs, and transformed it into our kanban.

Our kanban look very different from those you'll find at a Toyota factory (*see page 22*). But we designed them for the same purpose: communicate the who, what, where, and when for everyone on the team. The only difference is that we were moving the right *people* to the right place at the right time, instead of parts and products.

Our kanban is divided into different horizontal rows (swim lanes) corresponding to the different dental providers. An arrow pointing to the hygienist lane, for example, means that the patient needs to be seen by the hygienist. The resulting pattern of arrows reflects the *path of care* that the patient will follow. But the patient never moves; we come to the patient.

It's critical to remember that the kanban is NOT filled out ahead of time. This is NOT "assembly line dentistry." The coordinated schedule is developed as each provider ensures that something value-added is always being done for the patient … no gaps!

The first swim lane belongs to the front desk assistant. We see the appointment time, the time when the patient actually arrived and signed in (SI), and the time the patient was brought back (BB) to the patient room. Our goal is to bring patients back at the same time they sign in (SI = BB). Each provider has a swim lane with two times recorded: time given (TG) is the time that the provider receives the patient's kanban; time needed (TN) is the time that the provider is needed to begin his or her part of the treatment. Each provider adds information as to who the next provider should be, what they need to do, and when they can or should begin their part of the treatment. This determines which services get "pulled" next.

When a provider gets a kanban, he or she must assess whether the designated TN is possible. If it is, there will be no gaps in the treatment. If it's not, then the flow manager helps the provider meet the schedule, finds another provider, or changes the sequence. In any case, the patient's treatment continues uninterrupted.

Patient Treatment Kanban

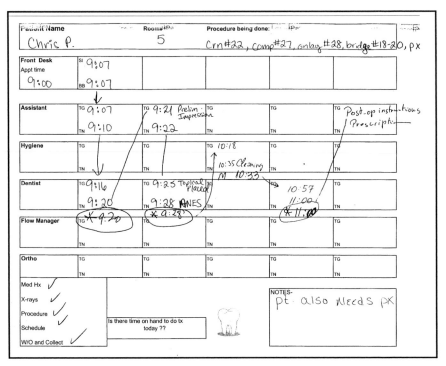

In the example above, our patient had an appointment time of 9 a.m.; actually arrived, signed in, and was brought back at 9:07. The kanban and the patient's treatment then progress as follows:

1. The assistant is given a kanban at 9:07 to begin her work at 9:10. She begins the patient's treatment at 9:10.

2. The dentist receives the kanban at 9:16, showing that he is needed at 9:20. The dentist sees the patient for the first time at 9:20.

3. The assistant is given the kanban at 9:21, asking her to do a preliminary impression at 9:22. The impression is made at 9:22 and the assistant numbs the patient's gum for the next step in the treatment.

4. The dentist is given the kanban at 9:25, telling him that he is needed at 9:28. He arrives at 9:28, anesthetizes the patient, and begins treatment.

5. The hygienist receives her kanban at 10:18, requesting that she begin cleaning the patient's teeth at 10:35. She begins the cleaning at 10:33.

6. The dentist receives the kanban at 10:57 to begin the final segment of treatment at 11:00. The dentist begins treatment at 11:00, as soon as the hygienist has completed the patient's cleaning.

7. The assistant receives the kanban, telling her that she must be prepared to provide post-op instructions and prescriptions for the patient when today's treatment is completed.

Each provider was able to meet their TN, the flow manager did not have to get involved, and the patient received four dental procedures and a cleaning in a single four-hour appointment.

We actually plan our day in the morning meeting, knowing that the schedule is likely to change because of factors beyond our control. However, once we start treating patients, we shift our attention to what to do next so that only the next move is important.

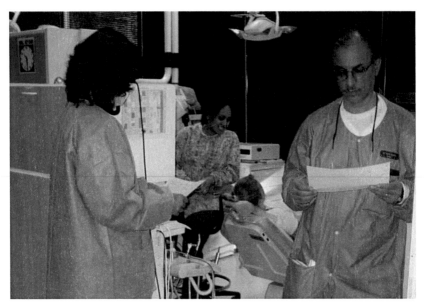

Dr. Bahri and hygienist Rosa Martinez using their kanban to see where and when they are needed next.

The flow manager orchestrates our successive "next moves" for the entire workday. Her main tool is the mighty kanban. It synchronizes more precisely than any computer program I know, and it is simple. It also offers the additional advantage of mapping the flow of each patient's treatment—studying the different charts at a later date might reveal some hidden patterns in our value streams. Who knows?

In addition to using the kanban, we created a system of visual signals for dentists, hygienists, and flow managers. A red card posted at a patient room is a dentist's or hygienist's method of alerting flow managers that they need extra help to get back on schedule. If a dental assistant is free, the flow manager asks her to help where needed. If all the assistants are busy, the flow manager helps; she is also cross-trained. Green cards hanging outside of patient rooms indicate that the dentists/hygienists are "on time," but most importantly, the patient's treatment is flowing.

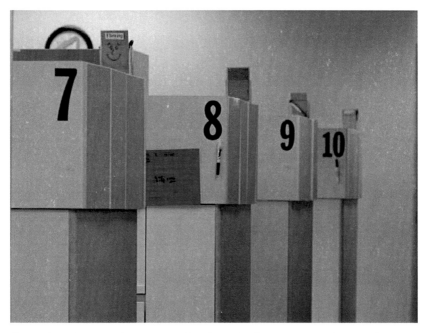

The red card atop patient room 8 signals to the flow manager that help is needed to stay on schedule.

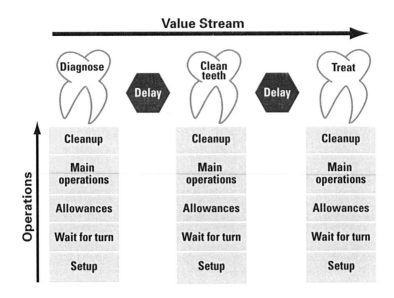

Value Stream

Diagnose — Delay — Clean teeth — Delay — Treat

Operations:
- Cleanup
- Main operations
- Allowances
- Wait for turn
- Setup

Delay: Anything preventing complete treatment in a single visit (additional appointments required)

Cleanup: Removing any materials from previous patients or procedures in preparation for the next patient/procedure

Main operations: Providing value-creating treatment/services

Allowances: Incidental work but necessary to support the main operations (e.g., moving or maintaining infrequently used equipment between rooms, rest, or personal hygiene breaks, etc.)

Wait for turn: Slowdown in the planned treatment (e.g., unavailable equipment, providers, necessary processing time such as waiting for materials to set or dry, etc.)

Setup: Preparing the needed equipment and supplies to provide treatment

Before 2005, we realized that the only time we were creating value was when we were doing our "main operations" where we delivered a service that moved a patient's treatment forward to completion. We also realized that all of the other things we did outside of these operations was waste and had to be reduced until they were eliminated. This helped us to focus our improvement efforts, but the overall experience of the patient did not change dramatically and neither did the capacity of the practice.

Our "trek" in 2005 allowed us to put all of the pieces of the puzzle together. It was like someone finally gave us the cover of the jigsaw puzzle as a guide. We realized that the treatment of the patient is our *value stream* made up of a series of *operations*. A value stream is made up of *all the actions—both value-creating and nonvalue-creating—required to deliver a service from the time a customer (or patient) orders it to the time it is completed*. In the diagram at left, the value stream moves horizontally while the operations flow vertically into each value-stream step. We saw that we had been spending all of our time and improvement efforts on getting rid of waste in the operations, while ignoring the reasons for delays *between* value-stream steps.

> Having a flow manager has made my life so much easier because I'm told where to go. You can see it two different ways … that somebody is telling the doctor where to go, but the way I see it, I don't have to worry about whether or not patients are waiting … I can focus on the work more. And if the patient requests another procedure, all I have to do is ask the flow manager.
>
> — Dr. Komal Relan, DMD
> Associate Dentist

We defined these delays as being any time the patient had to make a new appointment between steps in the treatment value stream—in other words, any interruption in the flow of treatment to the patient. So until we got rid of the reasons for these delays, our vision of one-patient flow was impossible.

We're able to easily switch from procedure to procedure rather than running around the office, looking for certain things, switching back and forth.

— Indira "Ida" Imsirovic
Expanded Duties Dental Assistant

Finally, we began to focus on eliminating waste in operations that made a difference! We identified and eliminated waste like long setup times and long distances between dentist and hygienist rooms, eliminating much of the delays between the different operations.

But the highest peak that we conquered was breaking down the barriers between functions—between dentists and hygienists. When this happened it was like being touched by an angel! It was magical because everything and everyone was working in a synchronized way with the patient at the center. We were finally flowing as a practice—not perfectly—but flowing, nonetheless.

So what does it mean for our practice to flow? The table below shows the results of our lean transformation in 2005.

Benefits of Applying Lean Concepts in Dentistry

	Hrs/Week Available to Dentists	Patient's Time for Complete Treatment	Hygienists	Assistants	Dentists	Patient Rooms
2005	77 hrs	99 days	3	5	3	10
2006	140 hrs	38 days	2	3	3	6
2007	140 hrs	12 days	2	3	3	6
2008	140 hrs	10 days	2	3	3	6
Results/ Improvement 2005 to 2008	+82%	+90%	+33%	+40%	--	+40%

Lean Definitions in Manufacturing and Dentistry

In Manufacturing

In Dentistry

Cycle Time
The time required to produce a part or complete a process, as timed by actual measurement.

We define **cycle time** as the time it takes to complete an operation like a dental cleaning, a root canal, or a crown.

Delays
Any time that value is not being immediately created in a product, with "value-creating" defined as what you do to a product at any step in the process that makes it more valuable in the eyes of the customer.

Delays represent anything that hinders the smooth flow of treatment. One form of delays hurts efficiency more than any other—treatment in multiple visits. The most efficient and economical treatment, for the dentist and the patient alike, is that which is finished on the exam day.

Just-In-Time (JIT)
A system of production that makes and delivers just what is needed, just when it is needed, and just in the amount needed.

We think of **JIT** as *making an appointment between a task and its providers*. If we know when a task needs to be performed and how long it takes, we're able to calculate the optimal time to start preparing for it.

We try to direct a care provider (dentist, hygienist, or assistant) to arrive at the patient's patient room exactly when the previous provider has finished the preceding treatment step. To coordinate their efforts we use the service kanban. This synchronization requires flexibility and precision.

Flexibility comes from cross-training and the willingness of the team members to take on various tasks as needed. *Precision*, on the other hand, comes from utilizing the information about the changes in demand as it comes, then changing the schedule as close to the appointment as is practical.

Kanban
A kanban is a signaling device that gives authorization and instructions for the production or withdrawal (conveyance) of items in a pull system. The term is Japanese for "sign" or "signboard."

We use 2 types of **kanban**:
- A paper *service kanban* to request the services of the different providers, directing them to where they are needed, at the time they are needed, and indicating to them what they are needed for.
- A simple *supplies kanban*. For example, the container of anesthetic carpules, for example, is utilized as a kanban to trigger reordering of anesthetics. Once the container is emptied in the patient room, it is given to the person in charge of ordering. She uses the information on the container to place the new order. She won't discard the old container until she receives the new one.

In Manufacturing	In Dentistry

Lead Time

The time it takes one piece to move all the way through a process or a value stream, from start to finish. Envision timing a marked part as it moves from beginning to end.

Lead Time is the time elapsed from the moment a patient calls for an appointment to the moment his or her mouth is totally healthy. We try to continuously reduce it by eliminating waste/nonvalue-adding activity.

Leveling

Leveling the type and quantity of production over a fixed period of time. This enables production to efficiently meet customer demands while avoiding batching, and results in minimum inventories, capital costs, manpower, and production lead time through the whole value stream.

Leveling means balancing load and capacity by distributing procedures evenly throughout the schedule, according to takt time.

Leveling the most frequent and repetitive procedure (dental cleanings) allows us to schedule the remaining appointments by patient rather than procedure.

Overproduction

Producing more, sooner, or faster than is required by the next process. Ohno considered over-production to be the most grievous form of waste because it generates and hides other wastes, such as inventories, defects, and excess transport.

Overproduction happens infrequently in direct patient treatment during which we are treating one tooth at a time. When patients leave the office we no longer can work on their teeth, so we are less likely to overproduce.

Accessory functions, however, are more likely to generate overproduction. A few examples: setups for patients who don't show up for appointments, printing patient forms before they are needed, obtaining insurance authorization for a "no-show" patient that then requires yet another authorization for the rescheduled appointment.

Processing

Any activity that transforms a product to something more valuable to the customer.

In terms of **processing**, whenever the patient is being treated, value is being created from the point of view of the customer.

The main question is: What is happening to our patients' mouths at every moment of the appointment from when they enter our reception area to when they are dismissed?

Four answers are possible: the tooth is processed (being treated); it's waiting or being delayed; it's being inspected; or it's being transported.

In Manufacturing	In Dentistry

Rightsizing Containers

Processing equipment that is highly capable, easy to maintain (and therefore available to produce whenever needed), quick to changeover, easy to move, and designed to be installed in small increments of capacity to facilitate capital and labor linearity.

We use **rightsizing of containers** to ensure the *largest variety of instruments and supplies* around the dental practitioner with the goal of reducing setup times—or even eliminating them altogether—if possible.

We put *small bins* in the cabinets around the dentist and the assistant. We divide them into *small compartments measured to fit the size of the materials they hold*. Small quantities of a wide variety of products are placed *within reach* of the operating teams, allowing them to perform around 90% of the usual dental procedures, without having to change setups.

Setup Reduction (Single Minute Exchange of Die, or SMED)

A process for changing over production equipment from one part number to another in as little time as possible. SMED refers to the target of reducing changeover times to a single digit, or less than 10 minutes.

Key insights about setup reduction, developed in the 1950s and 1960s, included separating *internal setup operations*—which can be done only when a machine is stopped (such as inserting a new die)—from *external operations* that can be performed while the machine is running (such as transporting the new die to the machine), and then converting internal setup operations to external operations.

Setup reduction is very important for the practice of dentistry. We used to batch similar procedures, such as crowns or fillings or veneers, in one appointment because different procedures necessitate different setups. To combine the different procedures in one appointment, we had to reduce the setup time, eliminating it whenever possible.

Internal setup operations can be done only when the patient is not in the room. *External* setup operations can be performed while the patient is still in the chair.

A *patient turnover setup* is required when switching treatment between two different patients. Traditionally, the problem is resolved in dentistry by preparing different patient rooms for different patients, multiplying the number of rooms for the same dentist.

A *procedure turnover setup* is required when we switch procedures on the same patient. While patients are in the dental chair, we need to be able to switch from a root canal, for instance, to a crown procedure without having to stop and change setups.

We must find ways to prepare external setups as close to the appointment time as is practical to avoid any waste created by situations such as canceled appointments.

In Manufacturing	In Dentistry
Standardized Work Establishing precise procedures for each operator's work in a production process, based on three elements: 1. Takt time, which is the *rate* at which products must be made in a process to meet customer demand 2. The precise work *sequence* in which an operator performs tasks within takt time 3. The standard *inventory*, including units in machines, required to keep the process operating smoothly	To **standardize work** methods, we distinguish between standard operations and standard processes. Standard operations relate to how a specific operation like a crown or root canal is performed. These individual operation standards are left to the discretion of each dentist. The heart of lean is the process, not the operation. Therefore, we have worked very diligently to standardize the sequence/ process of treatment. We standardized the room layouts, materials, and instruments. However, we needed to respect each dentist's preferences for treatment and technique choices. We place common materials in fixed bins in an identical setting across all patient rooms. We then place individual dentists' materials in movable containers so they can move them between the rooms.
Supermarket The location where a predetermined standard inventory is kept to supply downstream processes. Supermarkets ordinarily are located near the supplying process to help that process see customer usage and requirements. Each item in a supermarket has a specific location from which a material handler withdraws products in the precise amounts needed by a downstream process.	In our practice, we use two types of **supermarkets**: A *visible supermarket* used for dental supplies is practical and visible in the form of a cart, movable among the 10 patient rooms to resupply small dental material bins. In the bins, the materials are always available to the dentist and assistant at the moment of treatment, making it unnecessary to set up new materials when we are switching procedures. In a service environment, we also use an *invisible* (abstract) *supermarket* for some supporting procedures, such as the verification of insurance benefits before the patient's actual appointment time. To be safe, the insurance manager might gather this information 2–3 hours ahead of an appointment even though it usually takes only 30 minutes to get it. The data sitting in her computer 2–3 hours before it is needed is a virtual information supermarket. It's waiting to be used when needed. It's close to JIT, but not quite ... Any earlier than this and it could be overproduction, preventing the assistant from performing value-adding work because she would be busy verifying insurance benefits before this step is actually needed.

In Manufacturing	In Dentistry
Takt Time The available production time divided by customer demand.	A procedure's **takt time** is found by dividing the number of minutes worked during a certain time period by the number of times patients order that procedure (e.g., teeth cleaning or root canal) during that same period. By comparing takt time to a procedure's cycle time we could level the schedule and determine the number of people needed to perform the task. For example, because the cycle time needed to perform a dental cleaning (21 minutes) was shorter than its takt time (26 minutes) the process flowed smoothly. If the cycle time for a cleaning was longer than its takt time, we would have needed more hygienists and more-complex scheduling efforts for a timely cleaning delivery.

Part II: Leading the Transformation

Part I focused on what changed at Bahri Dental Group in pursuit of one-patient flow from the perspective of the patient and staff. In this section, Dr. Bahri shifts to discussing the how of the transformation. He describes how lean concepts changed his own definition of a leader. He also focuses on the critical importance of the new lean "mental model" that he first had to define and then introduce to the rest of the organization.

The remainder of the section describes the role that Dr. Bahri played in carefully introducing the required changes in thinking and behavior in the practice and the keys to sustaining these changes over the long term.

Becoming a Change Leader

Until recently, I didn't think that the lean transformation we deployed had much to do with my leadership. We were just doing what we had to do to improve patient care. I never thought of myself as a leader, nor was I aware that we were creating a new management system in the field of dentistry. Through the whole journey we were attempting to figure out which lean principles were useful to us and how to implement them.

Early in my career, the basic elements of leadership seemed simple to me: a constant goal and a method by which to reach it. Implementation should then become a matter of good communication and effective interaction with my staff. This was something that could be refined with experience, I thought. But many years of intense thinking proved that identifying a specific goal was not so simple to achieve. At that time, I did not even have a vision for my practice, mainly because I didn't understand the dental market and its needs.

I started experimenting with different approaches to find out which generated a more favorable response from both staff and patients. At times I was results-oriented and offered financial incentives to my hygienists for reaching financial production goals. When this approach created problems, I switched to focusing on customer service, then to promoting cosmetic services. We focused on innovation and technology for a time, and also tried adding accessory services like teeth whitening, specialized tooth brushes, and halitosis treatments to attract more patients.

I thought about encouraging employees to work harder and faster, hoping to solve the patient-waiting problem. Motivating employees with financial incentives and praise, or telling them how disappointed I was when they did not reach the efficiency and productivity goals of the practice, not only failed to provide tangible results but also exhausted me and my staff.

If employees need constant leadership, then leaders also need to be constantly motivated. Otherwise, how can they transmit their energy to the people they're supposed to lead? Deciding what project or idea to try next depended on what book I was reading at the time. If I came across an idea that I thought would be useful to the practice, I would discuss it with my staff and try it out, but ideas and projects were scattered, coming from different sources without a clear goal in mind.

Identifying the New Mental Model

Leading change during the lean transformation was much easier for me than during the years preceding it.

When I first read *Lean Thinking* and began learning about process waste and focused on eliminating it, "waste" became the buzz word at the office. Some employees got excited about the idea and started seeing waste everywhere. I could see that we were making progress toward our vision of process excellence, but again, while I was learning about lean, my leadership was not focused on a specific goal. I soon realized more efforts were needed on my part as a leader for the lean transformation to take root and be successful. At no time was I confident that we would ever see the much anticipated results we hoped lean would deliver, but I always believed in what Thomas Edison said: *"Many of life's failures are people who did not realize how close they were to success when they gave up."*

What I came to understand is that a lean transformation based on one-patient flow must take place in a business before the managing team starts focusing on *kaizen*—eliminating waste in the individual operations. In this sense, lean has given me a good reference system to clearly decide which ideas and practices are useful and which are unnecessary, based on whether or not they enhance or hinder the advancement of one-patient flow in dental treatment. Because this idea has proved itself to be so pivotal in our practice, I have included it in the definitions of *waste* and *improvement* when communicating lean principles with my staff. Today we define waste as "any activity that does not contribute to one-patient flow," and improvement as "any activity that shortens lead time through one-patient flow and just-in-time practices."

Establishing these base definitions was a breakthrough for my staff and me, but it had an even more profound impact on how I led my practice. Until I adopted lean as my management system, I was unable to settle on a vision for my practice. One-patient flow and short lead times came to mean much more than rapidly finishing one job at a time; it meant that we were bringing patients back to full health very quickly, with fewer dental appointments and less disruption to their lives at work and at home. With lean, I found that we were able to provide patients with *better dental care faster*. By making treatment more convenient and less daunting, we consistently saw more patient compliance with treatment and therefore an overall improvement in health. It also simplified how to measure our performance. I realized that if *one-patient flow* and *lead-time reduction* were whole system efficiency measures, any other metric inside my management system could be improved by maintaining focus on just these two factors.

Introducing Change

The translation of lean principles into dentistry was a necessary and challenging step in the lean transformation project. Dissecting lean principles like leveling or takt time was a very lengthy task, and there were many times I felt overwhelmed. But if a principle went unsolved at first, I could not stop thinking about it until I discovered its meaning and significance for my business. Each lean principle went through three stages before it became part of our daily working life.

First, I had to learn about the principles and understand their meaning in a manufacturing context. They were very unfamiliar to me as a dentist. I read and reread lean books until I felt I understood each principle well enough to communicate it to my staff.

Second, I had to translate each principle into dental terms. I started by sharing specific principles with my staff, trying to describe what they meant for manufacturing and then explaining what I thought each meant when applied to dentistry. How I communicated specific principles depended on the circumstances of the moment. I did whatever seemed simplest at the time. Sometimes I would discuss them in a meeting with everyone. Sometimes I would talk to just one staff member, wanting to hear just one person's opinion. There were plenty of occasions when opinions differed from mine. Thinking things through with my staff was very helpful to me though, because I knew they saw opportunities for improvement in our work that I could not always see.

Lastly, we had to actually apply these lean principles to the practice. This was the most challenging step because it meant radically changing the way we did our jobs. It required us to change personal methods and behavior, so we moved forward carefully when implementing them. I found that people were usually willing to move ahead based on a very simple promise: if it doesn't work, we can always return to how we do it now. Just this assurance seemed to calm so many fears.

Also, it helped that we always started small, usually trying ideas with me, one hygienist, and one assistant at a time. Then we paused to analyze what did not go according to our plans and thought carefully about how we might want to do things next time. Then we tried again with a different patient, still involving the same dentist, hygienist, and assistant. In weekly meetings we communicated the progress of our work with the rest of our team, hoping to get them interested in our experiment. I preferred to wait until my staff pulled information from me by asking questions about our projects. Little by little new and improved procedures spread throughout the office to become part of our standard operations.

It was my job to make it clear to everyone that all of these minor and major changes were part of a new system focusing on one-patient flow. I also had to make sure that we all understood that we had gone through a logical set of steps to get there. The results were dramatic and no accident. I strongly believe that this realization gave all of us (especially me) a sense of control over our direction. There was renewed energy and hope for the future of the practice. The atmosphere at the office was totally different from the one preceding the transformation. The improvements were life changing. Everyone's way of doing business at the office had changed. Hygienists did not have their own dedicated rooms anymore; instead they shared the dentists' rooms. The insurance coordinator and treatment plan coordinator became patient care flow managers, and instead of spending their days behind their desks, they were now on the clinic floor, helping patients where treatment is administered, or as they say in lean manufacturing, at the *gemba*, meaning "actual place," as in where value-creating work actually occurs.[4]

Sustaining Lean Leadership

This is where we find ourselves now. Once the conditions for basic flow were established, the era of "radical change" applied to the whole business was over. The office atmosphere has since shifted so that it feels like the calm after the storm, or should I say, the calm after a big party.

4. *Lean Lexicon*, p. 25.

Some people say that for a team to stay motivated it needs to operate in emergency mode all the time. A hospital emergency room setting is frequently used as an example. In an emergency room, providers are focused on saving a patient's life and, therefore, have little time for bickering. But how could I create the atmosphere of an emergency room without also creating constant stress? I was driving home from work one evening when the answer came to me like a revelation. What brings us together and makes us most efficient is clearly seeing the current problems that stop us from achieving and maintaining one-patient flow. Once problems are clearly communicated among staff, the desire to eliminate them incites people to collectively take corrective action. Instead of me or other staff members generating ideas randomly, ideas started to build and flow logically from each other.

After this breakthrough we started discussing problems and discovering next steps together. Leading improvement became much easier once the process itself started to expose the steps in a natural sequence. In this way we've gone from big steps and celebrations to smaller continuous improvement steps. One may think leadership as we move into this continuous improvement phase is even more difficult to sustain, but it's actually just the opposite. We have matured together in the system. When presented with a problem, we think about it in very similar ways. We have a system to discuss problems and find solutions efficiently asking questions like:

- You would like to improve a process. What part of the process isn't working?
- What is your proposed countermeasure? What are its advantages and disadvantages?
- What other countermeasures have you thought of?

Such decisions are never-ending in an improvement culture and are much easier to make when evaluated against clear criteria. In our case this criterion is simply one-patient flow. If a proposal helps promote it we call it a good countermeasure; if it doesn't promote it, it's reworked or discarded. Everyone understands why—decision accepted. In the same vein, cost reduction or improvements in only one area of the business or waste elimination in an isolated operation are just not enough. We need to reduce cost, eliminate waste, and facilitate one-patient flow all at the same time. We all understand "a good decision" in the same way. Rather than "selling" decisions, I'm either making decisions or asking my staff to decide using the same standard: one-patient flow.

When we identify an obstacle to one-patient flow, when we understand the need to eliminate it, and when our experiment demonstrates the benefits of its elimination, the whole staff becomes excited about spreading the new improvement throughout the business. We then give it some time to settle down. When it becomes part of our daily routine (standard work), our enthusiasm naturally diminishes, until we find the next obstacle to one-patient flow.

A lot of times, I'm not going to lie, all of us ... if Dr. Bahri says something, we're like "Oh gosh, no. What is this going to turn out to be?!" but once we see it, we think, "Why didn't we do this before?" It's the fear of change is what it is.

— Christine Catlin
Insurance Manager

My job is to enthusiastically lead these "waves of improvement," sometimes as a player and other times as a coach from the sidelines. I find the emotions of glory and defeat in business to be no different from those in a team sport. It's easy to be an effective coach because the basic elements of leadership are embedded in the PDCA process itself. Although reward programs can sometimes encourage people to improve faster, we have not needed them this far to get our team excited about creating the next wave of lean improvements.

Like perfection, one-patient flow with every patient, on every visit is unreachable. Like true north, however, it gives me a direction to follow. Now that we know where the boat is going, we can almost set it on auto-pilot. If I had to describe this process in a metaphor, I would say that instead of having to walk in front of my people to constantly find where to go, I can take the time to walk next to them, excitedly exploring the problems and possible countermeasures along the way. Implementation essentially means asking your employees to continually change their lives at work, and be happy about it. Lean has given me the practical tool that I needed to keep myself and my staff constantly intellectually stimulated. Our commitment to uncovering problems and encouraging solutions has become more important to the business and our employees than any other skill we've developed.

I predict that one-patient flow will remain the goal for the rest of my career, allowing me to create Dr. W. Edwards Deming's first principle, constancy of purpose. This simplifies life for my staff and shows our patients with every visit that they really are the most important part of Bahri Dental Group.

Part III: Discovering the Principles of Lean Leadership

So far Dr. Bahri has addressed how lean concepts, tools, and practices became part of his growing dental practice and described the dramatic impact of focusing on one-patient flow as Bahri Dental Group's guiding operating philosophy. But what leadership principles should a lean leader live by on a daily basis?

Here in Part III, Dr. Bahri shares the principles that he has found to be most helpful over the last 17 years, along with some of the sources of his knowledge and inspiration.

Become a Lean Leader by Focusing on Purpose, Process, and People

When I think about the principles that have helped me become more of a lean leader, I've found it useful to organize them into three areas: *Purpose, Process,* and *People.* I learned this from Jim Womack who suggests that it is the combination of all three that makes the Toyota Management System so powerful because it includes a clear and universally understood *purpose* dedicated to solving customer problems, supported by lean *processes* that are designed, performed, and improved by engaged *people* with fulfilling work.

This sounds so simple, yet it's very hard to achieve. My challenge as a lean leader is to live by these three principles every day so that the whole system works. The principles in this section are the ones that I have found to be most important in my own development as a lean leader.

Purpose

My first responsibility as a lean leader is to create a clear and motivating purpose that guides the direction of our practice and the behavior of everyone who works in it. If we are really practicing lean, this purpose must be based on the value that we are delivering to our customers. If we can clearly define that value, then this creates the "compass" that tells us when we are on course and when we need to do a course correction or improvement. Without this, it would be impossible for our organization to continuously improve. But there is another kind of guiding purpose that only a lean leader can provide —organizational values. These are the "rules of the road" that everyone (from me to our newest employee) follows when making decisions. I must make these values clear to the entire organization and then hold everyone accountable (especially myself) for living them everyday. How did I define my own purpose? Just as importantly, how did we become "purpose driven"?

Define "True North"

The purpose of my career is to make high quality dental services accessible to as many people as possible. When I say, *accessible to as many people as possible*, I do not mean my patients only. I deeply believe that healthcare professionals are morally obligated to improve healthcare systems in their offices, in their communities, in their countries, and in the world. It doesn't matter how we participate necessarily, as long as we're contributing.

In dentistry, we do all that we can to ensure that patients have their teeth for as long as they need them. We satisfy the functional criteria (eating and speaking) as well as the aesthetic criteria. Clinical care is only one part of dental services though. We have come to carefully consider other aspects of the patient experience from the moment our patients call the office to when we treat their teeth.

Accessible does not only mean affordable. It is true that some people have financial constraints that prevent them from seeking dental care, but there are other constraints as well. Often patients cannot take time away from work or their families. Making appointments, receiving patients, explaining treatment, presenting patients with financial options, and accommodating patients' schedules are other services we provide on a regular basis. We want to provide high-quality customer care just like any other service company does. Saying I didn't know how to do this is an understatement; I didn't even know the full range of services that touched the customer.

To find out, I went on a long research journey. I looked at management systems outside dentistry just to see how other industries were utilizing their resources. I read everything available to a novice. The work of authors like Stephen Covey, Masaaki Imai, Tom Peters, Peter Senge, Michael Hammer, Phil Crosby, Peter Drucker, Michael Gerber, Carl Sewell, and Michael LeBoeuf all became familiar.

I also talked to my colleagues about management, asking them what knowledge and insights they could offer. To share this knowledge of how to reach true north, my team and I have spent several months, sometimes years, trying to apply each book's concepts. Although we have rarely been able to adopt all of them, a good number of our discoveries over the years have become permanent components of our management vision.

Put the Customer First

Thank God for Joe.

Joe was the supplier who helped me set up my first practice. He had 40 years of experience in dentistry. I asked him a question over lunch one day: "If you had to think of one marketing idea in dentistry, what would it be?"

"If you needed to go to a wedding tomorrow and wanted your teeth cleaned, you could probably call all of the dentists in Jacksonville and still won't find one able to give you an appointment," Joe said. "If you can clean people's teeth when they request it, you will get a lot of business."

The possibility of doing this never occurred to me! To provide the kind of flexibility he spoke about, I immediately hired an additional hygienist with an open schedule. She took patients who needed cleanings on a short notice and began to treat more patients per day. Although we eventually changed our approach to scheduling in pursuit of one-patient flow, this was important because it was the first time we really began thinking about our work from the patient's perspective.

Then in 1993, I read Sam Walton's book, *Made in America*. It made me realize that besides understanding what's important to the customer, you also must be willing to do what's right by the customer every time. This was at the heart of Sam Walton's business strategy. He looked for merchandise at greatly reduced prices and passed on nearly all of the resulting gain to the customer. "For my whole career in retail, I have stuck to one guiding principle," he wrote. "The secret to successful retailing is to give your customers what they want."[5]

5. Walton, Sam. *Made in America*. New York: Bantam Books, 1993. p. 220.

> The focus is on the patient. The patient doesn't care who's doing what, where everything is coming from. It's what's making it easier for you to treat them and give them what they need: fast results and quality care.
>
> — RynaEllen Gwinn
> Expanded Duties
> Dental Assistant

Walton's unwavering commitment to providing as much value as he could was very inspiring. As health-care providers, our first obligation to our patients is to provide the right treatment while avoiding mistakes. But how could we, in dentistry, benefit from the ideas of *making the customer number one* and *giving them what they want?*

We know our customers want flexibility; they want to be able to make appointments on short notice. How do we change our habits so that we can provide this to them? And what else do they want?

Focus First on Reliability and Responsiveness

I found Berry and Parasuraman's book, *Marketing Services*, to be very helpful in looking at our services from the patient's perspective. In one study they asked more than 1,900 customers from five different industries to rate the relative importance of the five dimensions that influence customers' assessment of service quality by allocating 100 points among them.

The five dimensions ranked as follows:
1. Reliability (32 points)
2. Responsiveness (22 points)

3. Empathy (16 points)
4. Assurance (19 points)
5. Tangibles (11 points)

"Reliability is the essence of service quality,"[6] they concluded. I thought reliable service would require competent staff and sound business processes, so we started working on both. We dedicated every Thursday afternoon to training on both the technical side of procedures and deepening our understanding of lean and other ways to continuously improve. Because we had a small staff, training was not difficult, but required a lot of discipline to stick to this commitment. Especially as a practice is getting established it can be very tempting to fill every available hour with an appointment. Since then, finding time for training has been an ongoing process, happening at every open opportunity.

Pursue Quality and Productivity with Equal Passion

In the earlier part of my career, when I practiced dentistry in a batch mode, I found that *quality* worked in opposition with *accessibility* and *productivity*. The predominant thinking at the time was that dentists could either be productive or provide high quality service, but could not do both. Because my goal has always been to make dental care accessible to patients, for a time I thought I should work faster to increase productivity. The only problem with working faster is that you are more likely to make mistakes.

---

6. Berry, Leonard L. and A. Parasuraman. *Marketing Services: Competing Through Quality.* New York: Free Press, 1991. p. 16.

In contrast, quality leaders agreed that improving quality was the most efficient way of doing business. Deming said it in *Out of the Crisis*.[7] Phil Crosby went so far as to call his book *Quality Is Free*. In *The Machine That Changed the World*, Womack and Jones studied the relationship between productivity and quality in many manufacturing plants scattered around the world. They concluded that companies that practice in batch-and-queue mode could have either high quality or high productivity, but could not possibly have both. They showed real examples of companies that were able to stay productive while still providing high quality products. Finding a way to achieve both goals was very important to me, especially working in health care.

I was first introduced to Dr. Deming's teachings by Michael Dagher, a friend and MD who managed the emergency room at Memorial Hospital in Jacksonville. I was very frustrated with employee problems and asked him for advice. Our discussion led me to explore a whole new management world.

When I asked Michael for a reference, he recommended that I read Mary Walton's book, *The Deming Management Method*, because it was simple enough for me to understand. It introduced me to SPC, which I started applying in my office. This was not easy without guidance, but little by little we gained some understanding of the tools, collected and analyzed data, and corrected what Deming called *special causes* of problems and defects. Special causes are *events that are unusual or unpredictable*. These are different from *common causes*, which *result from normal variation in a stable system*.

---

7. Deming, W. Edwards. *Out of the Crisis*. Cambridge, MA: MIT Press, 1982. p. 309.

Minimize Lead Time and Maximize Flow to Increase Capacity

With his book, *The Toyota Production System,* Taiichi Ohno introduced the Toyota Produciton System to the world. This book is full of good information, but I focused on just a few ideas that set lean apart from other management systems:

Reduce lead time: "All we are doing is looking at the time line from the moment the customer gives us an order to the point when we collect the cash. And we are reducing that time line by removing the nonvalue-added wastes."[8]

Establish flow: "Unless one completely grasps this method of doing work so that things will flow, it is impossible to go right into the kanban system when the time comes."[9] I added that one-piece flow is the ideal condition. A basic principle in the pull system says that all a worker needs to know from a scheduling standpoint, is what to do next. Extrapolating to dentistry, I thought changes are bound to happen to the schedule we create each day. The flow manager was our response to this reality.

Increase capacity: "Change the manner in which things flow and change the manner in which you arrange your storage, and you will discover within a month that you can do whatever you have been saying you cannot do. Not only can you do it, but you will be left a little extra change after paying the bill. In fact you can even eliminate some of the processes!"[10] To increase capacity, I realized all we had to do was change the operations sequence and the way we stored supplies.

---

8. Ohno, Taiichi. *The Toyota Production System: Beyond Large-Scale Production.* New York: Productivity Press, 1988. p. ix.

9. Ibid., p. 33.

10. Japan Management Association. *Kanban Just-In-Time at Toyota: Management Begins at the Workplace.* New York: Productivity Press, 1986. p. 9.

Understand and Treat the Organization as a System

In 1994, I stumbled upon a book by Peter Senge, *The Fifth Discipline*, in which he describes "five new component technologies that are gradually converging to innovate learning organizations."[11] He describes four core disciplines to building the learning organization: personal mastery, mental models, shared vision, and team learning. His fifth discipline "*integrates the other disciplines, fusing them into a coherent body of theory and practice*," called systems thinking.[12]

This was my first introduction to thinking about my business as a whole. Later, I would apply this concept to my practice by breaking down functional barriers between the different functions at the dental office—front desk, hygienist, dentist, financial manager, insurance coordinator, etc. It was only then that I stopped thinking of the different areas of my practice as separate "profit centers," but rather as parts of a whole system.

The MIT beer distribution simulation that Senge describes in his book was especially helpful. This was a role-playing simulation developed at MIT in the 1960s to show the advantages of taking an integrated approach to managing a supply chain. Instead of integration, the players in the simulation showed erratic behavior that Senge partially attributes to the presence of *delays in the feedback processes*. These delays make it difficult to understand the cause-and-effect relationship of one's actions. To improve the decision-making process it becomes critical to eliminate delays in the feedback processes that occur.

How does that apply to dentistry? Simple. If we find a cavity while examining a mouth, we have the information about the condition of that tooth fresh in our mind. Therefore, we can treat the tooth with

11. Senge, Peter. *The Fifth Discipline*. New York: Broadway Business, 2006. p. 6.
12. Ibid., p. 12.

minimal risks of making mistakes. On the contrary, if we delay the treatment for a few months, we might forget some of the details, even after writing good notes in the patient's chart. We might have to double-check our diagnosis and reassess the tooth. By focusing on this simple idea of avoiding delays—for example, between diagnosis and treatment—we were able to reduce lead times and get that much closer to achieving one-patient flow.

Another cause of the chaotic decision-making process in the beer game was the lack of communication between the different players and parts of the system. Although we were operating within a smaller system, we experienced this same lack of communication, especially as we increased our flexibility in scheduling. We largely eliminated this problem by developing the service kanban described earlier.

Pursue Operational Excellence; Growth Will Follow

Once we improved our work processes and began seeing the benefits of TQM, lean, and a whole-system approach to management, we needed to learn how to efficiently manage the large number of patients we had. Early on, the answer felt obvious to me: add more staff. Every time we had too much work to handle, I thought I should add a staff member. This was my solution, but the more people I had on staff, the more complicated it became to manage them. I then became as overwhelmed with staff management as with patient management.

I always wanted to have a large office with several providers, while still keeping the highest standards in treatment and service excellence. To reach my goal I knew that I needed to build a well-trained, competent staff.

The most frequent advice I have encountered in my readings was to create a vision for my business, then communicate it to my staff, and find the systems that would allow us to reach the vision. *The Discipline of Market Leaders* by Treacy and Wiersema helped me to clarify the context in which I wanted to place my vision ideas:

> In the same way that customers cluster into three different categories … companies cluster into distinctively different value disciplines … By *operational excellence*, we mean providing customers with reliable products or services at competitive prices, delivered with minimal difficulty or inconvenience. By *product leadership*, we mean providing products that continually redefine the state of the art. And by *customer intimacy*, we mean selling the customer a total solution, not just a product or service … Not choosing [a value discipline] means ending up in the middle. It means hybrid operating models that are neither here nor there, and that consequently cause confusion, tension, and loss of energy.[13]

We have clearly chosen the operational excellence route. Of course, we will continue to bring innovative products and complete dental solutions to our patients, but operational excellence will set us apart. Any practice can incorporate new treatments and technologies— practices in very competitive markets are constantly looking for "new and improved" services to hold onto existing patients and attract new ones. But if we can treat our patients with the latest technology *and* provide them with more flexible scheduling and a no-waiting treatment process, who can compete with us?

13. Treacy, Michael and Fred Wiersema. *The Discipline of Market Leaders: Choose Your Customers, Narrow Your Focus, Dominate Your Market*. New York: Perseus Books, 1995. p. 45.

Process

If our purpose sets our direction, our processes determine how we get there. Unlike the days when I used to focus only on results— "I don't care how you get there as long as you deliver the numbers"— as a lean leader, I must be equally concerned with results and methods.

By focusing on both the *why* behind the work (purpose/strategy) and *how* people do their work (processes), lean leaders encourage learning at all levels within the organization. I must demonstrate "process thinking" when I create plans (e.g., What documented process are we going to put in place to achieve our goal?) and solve problems, (e.g., What in our process caused this problem? What in our process must we change?)

This helps us to become a "learning organization" because all plans are actually experiments. We then use problem-solving to analyze the results. This process thinking is a way for everyone to focus on fixing problems through learning, rather than on fixing the blame.

It's about *why*, not *who*. This is a very different approach for most organizations, so it had to start with me. *How did I become a process thinker? How did we make process thinking a way of life?*

I did the numbers and my practice had increased by 30%. Partly because I was improving, but also because we changed the way we were doing things. I get very isolated doing my own thing, but he (Dr. Bahri) is able to step back and see the larger picture.

— Dr. Anjali Lueck, DMD
Associate Dentist

Be Equal Part Learner, Equal Part Teacher

I was 13 when my French teacher, a gentleman from Paris, came to congratulate me on my good performance in his class. I stood there wanting to tell him a lot of things but I was not confident in my language. While my teacher was pleased with the quality of my work, I still remember the feeling of not being able to express myself freely in another language.

On the last day of school that year before summer vacation, I made a decision: I was going to spend my vacation learning French to the best of my ability so that when I returned to school in the fall, I would be able to discuss whatever I wanted with my teacher without fear of making mistakes.

As soon as I got home I started reading one of my French novels, underlining the words I could not understand. When I had 10 words I would go to the dictionary and find their meaning. I wrote these definitions down next to the words. With these words I started building sentences, imagining how one day I was going to express my ideas in the classroom.

I had no interest that summer except to destroy that feeling of powerlessness I felt with my teacher that day. By the end of my summer, I was near fluent and felt confident speaking in French. This was probably my first experience learning something significant on my own without any guidance from a teacher. The taste of this success has kept me going; from that moment on I knew I needed to become responsible for my own learning.

My uncle Elias was also very successful at taking charge of his own learning. He studied English in school and learned French at home. As an adult he taught French and was a very passionate teacher. He did not see any difference between life at school and life at home. He constantly analyzed situations and facts, large issues like the Cold War, and small details like the origins of every word we used, how it evolved, and from what language.

To help his students learn, he would make poems out of French vocabulary words and give them a melody. I remember him telling me how surprised the principal was to hear his class singing. Uncle Elias instilled in me a love of learning and a desire to teach.

First Standardize, Then Improve

Michael Gerber's book, *The E-Myth* (or entrepreneurial myth), came just at the right time. My front desk assistant decided to go to nursing school just when I started feeling confident about her skills on the job. I became very nervous about training someone new to replace her. *The E-Myth* teaches you how to make a small business operate like a franchise. You begin by creating an organizational chart showing the different job functions in your organization. Starting with the simplest functions, you explain how each function is performed. New employees then are expected to follow these job descriptions exactly.

Taking advantage of the Thanksgiving holiday in 1995 and using Gerber's principles, I made a list of all the functions our new front desk assistant would need to perform. Then I created a procedure manual by printing computer screen shots of our dental software.

Next I connected the images with visual diagrams and flowcharts. I was not able to complete the whole manual in one weekend, but on her first day at work, our new assistant found enough information to perform her job properly.

This was probably our first serious attempt to work on the process itself in order to affect the end results. Unfortunately, during that time I still thought of standardization as something rigid, therefore impeding improvement. I did not like Gerber's thought of forbidding employees to improve work processes because I knew I needed my staff's suggestions. I wanted them to know that their ideas mattered and that they had the power to improve work for themselves and for their patients.

Once we began implementing lean, I started to consider standardization as the starting point for continuous improvement. For a while I was the only person writing "process standards forms," as we called them, and I grew discouraged having to repeatedly update them. But today all staff members prepare and update them. Like Toyota, we change our standard procedures to reflect our current best practices. We listen to employees and patients, and we improve our standards every time we find a better way to serve our patients' needs.

Build a Problem-Solving Culture
Living for 17 years during the Lebanese Civil War gave me numerous opportunities to find creative solutions to daily problems. Once I started analyzing specific situations though, I often felt the possibilities were so numerous that the whole process could easily become overwhelming and frustrating. I wanted to go back to dealing with life's

problems without deep analysis, but I knew I could not. Once again my Uncle Elias was a major influence. He taught me to isolate specific situations and dissect them almost scientifically. I had to become a scientific thinker to do more than just survive the chaos.

When it came to bringing my problem-solving thinking to Bahri Dental Group, I found Dr. Deming's teachings on continuous improvement to be very helpful. Dr. Deming's stature as one of the gurus of quality also gave me the confidence I needed to make scientific problem-solving part of our daily practice at the office. His PDCA cycle provided a simple and reliable approach. Since we have begun using PDCA, we have basically used it to overcome problems of any size. We use small PDCA cycles for small problems and large PDCA cycles for big problems. Seeing problems this way has transformed the way I looked at business and at life in general.

Making problem-solving a daily practice may sound like hard work—and in some ways it is—but I try to remind myself and my staff that solving problems can give us a satisfying sense of achievement and even be fun. In *Kaizen*, Imai tells us: "There is a saying among TQC (Total Quality Control) practitioners in Japan that problems are the '*keys to hidden treasures.*'"[14]

It is a totally different paradigm than what most managers are used to and instantly shifted my focus from avoiding any discussion about problems to trying to find as many problems as possible. Our culture shifted from a culture of blame to one of finding problems together and celebrating solutions. We started to think of problems as invisible obstacles standing between us and excellence.

---

14. Imai, Masaaki. *Kaizen: The Key to Japan's Competitive Success.* New York: McGraw-Hill, 1986. p. 163.

> He is the only doctor I've ever worked for who is receptive to what you have to say. You have to learn how to say it to him though ... You can't go in and say "Oh, this isn't working. This is awful. I hate this!" You have to go and say, "This is the problem. It's a problem because ... and could we try this instead?" And then he's always there for you.
>
> — Patricia Kelly
> Dental Hygienist

Today we understand that if we don't make problems visible, we won't be able to eliminate them and we won't be able to improve. When a problem is difficult enough to require some stretching of our mental or technical capabilities, it could lead the person attempting to solve it, I found, to what Mihály Csíkszentmihályi describes as the highly satisfying psychological "state of flow."

But you can't address problems until you find them and you can't find them until you can talk about them freely. During the early years of my practice, I thought it was better to focus on the positive things my staff did rather than the negative, hoping that people would abandon bad behaviors if I kept praising their good behavior every time I encountered it. This concept is very similar to the "catch them doing something right" idea in Ken Blanchard's *One Minute Manager*.[15]

When communicating with people, I always started by telling them something nice before giving them bad news or criticizing them. This concept makes sense and works in many situations, but there are drawbacks. I found it to work when dealing with behavior problems, but not systemic ones.

15. Blanchard, Kenneth and Spencer Johnson. *The One Minute Manager.* New York: William Morrow & Company, 1981. p. 36–37.

First, it encourages you to avoid talking about problems, hoping they will disappear once you emphasize the good things. But problems don't disappear and not surprisingly, my staff started ignoring the first part of our conversation during which I would tell them how valuable they were to the practice and how much I appreciated them. They were "waiting for the other shoe to drop." The predictability of the pattern undermined the trust factor between my staff and me.

The second drawback was that employees got used to the formula and began using it with each other. This weakened relationships rather than strengthened them because it was predictable and felt dishonest. After a while I chose to change styles, to skip the praise and go directly to the subject matter at hand. While problems aren't always pleasant to talk about, my staff has come to appreciate my honesty.

Cross-Train To Meet the Needs of the Patient

Looking back at our meeting notes from 1991, I saw that the seeds for cross-training were already planted long before we knew one-patient flow would be the goal. In July 1991, the chair-side assistants asked to be trained in front desk duties so they could help when needed. Their training started immediately. The front desk assistant created a visual signal to communicate with the chair-side assistants. If the phone rang and she was not able to answer it because she was busy with another patient, she would stand up. The chair-side assistants would know to answer that line for her.

In January 1992, the front desk assistant asked to be trained in surgical procedures so she could return the favor and help in the back when needed. She had graduated from a dental-assistants school a year earlier and her training was very easy. She gradually trained in other chair-side procedures until she could interchange positions with chair-side assistants.

In 1994, the chair-side assistants were ready to take full charge of their patients' needs including the front desk duties. Just mentioning what and how things needed to be done was no longer sufficient; assistants needed to be formally trained to avoid mistakes in handling their new tasks. We decided to dedicate every Thursday for cross-training only, without seeing any patients.

It was a big move, but it was better than seeing assistants and hygienists waiting for me and other dentists in the hallway. While I was treating my patients, they would chat amongst each other and rush me to finish whatever I was doing so that I could go attend to their patients. Patients could have been walked out and their insurance filed, but all of this had to wait. And at the hour when the dental appointments were over, patients from different rooms had to form a line at the front desk while one person processed all their paperwork. This was very inefficient.

The Thursday training sessions went very well, and the assistants learned most of what they needed. After a few years, the day-long training sessions were no longer necessary, so we shortened them to Friday afternoon sessions instead. When more doctors joined the practice in 2001, it became more difficult to stop work on patients and meet for cross-training. We replaced the Friday afternoons with daily 15-minute morning meetings to discuss improvements. To supplement these daily discussions, we used more on-the-job training. Most of the staff members were competent enough by then to make on-the-job training of new employees effective.

Create a Learning Environment Safe for Experimentation

Being made director of the dental school in Beirut during the early 1980s forced me to look for what other people were doing to keep their teams motivated and to manage their time and resources better. After managing the dental school for a couple years I felt the need to actively pursue whatever theories were available at that time.

For the five-year period I was in charge of directing the school, my colleagues and I often introduced new ideas and projects. As years went by I also noticed that certain systems implemented in the early years were either not working or were not adaptable to the growth of the school. The need for change became more pressing as time went by. But as in every organization, people had become comfortable in their positions so that when we tried to initiate changes, we encountered a lot of resistance. Simple things like checking in with a patient or performing a surgery, or moving a patient from a fillings department to the prosthodontics department were not so simple after all. People wanted to know who was in charge of each process at the time, and who would be in charge of each process after we changed them.

An illustration of a little change that we wanted to implement would be in the way we received and examined our patients on the first floor of the clinic in the diagnostics department. The department had four instructors; three had proposed a new process for receiving, examining, and coordinating the treatment planning for new patients, and one person, a veteran who had founded the department, was not ready to go forward with the new project. I went upstairs to meet with the rest of the group, and I asked everyone to explain their point of view.

Trying to break the ice, I looked at my friend and said, "You have three people desiring to try a project to see how it works. Would you be willing to let them try, and if it does not work we will revert back to the old ways?" He answered, "I would like to try, but I want to have it noted in the meeting report that I am against the project."

This approach worked like magic. After hours of deadlock, asking someone not to change his mind, but rather to give us a *chance* to try something new, and providing the reassurance that we would revert to old methods if necessary, proved to be a very efficient approach at softening people's positions and ultimately opening their minds to the possibility of change.

The key point I have found is to be genuine about it. If new methods don't work, then we have a decision to make. Do we evaluate the new methods once again or go back to what we had done originally? We've had to revert in a few instances, but in the overwhelming majority of cases, people prefer to re-evaluate the situation and think about what problems are preventing us from implementing our project. Then we find countermeasures that allow the improvement to happen.

In the end, my friend did not revert to the old way of doing things. After trying the new treatment methods, he even helped everybody tweak the different processes and make them better.

He's always studying, learning, and reading. I was looking for that ... I didn't want to stop learning just because I started working.

— Dr. Anjali Lueck, DMD
Associate Dentist

Communicate Clearly and Honestly With Patients

When I started my practice in Jacksonville, my accent was so heavy that my patients couldn't clearly understand me when I tried to explain their treatment plans. I often had to go into my office with my assistant and explain the treatment plan to her so that she could explain it to the patient. I remember listening to CNN in my car on the way to and from work and trying to repeat certain English words over and over, trying to mimic the news anchors' speech until I was able to speak so that my patients could understand me.

My practice was very slow at first. When I look back at my schedule, I see that I had one or two patients a day. For a long time I was even borrowing money from the bank to pay my rent and my employees. It was clear that I needed to attract more patients to the practice, so I learned marketing. After a few months, my patient base began to grow.

A new problem eventually arose. Although I was able to get patients through the door, I was not able to convince them of the treatment they needed, and therefore, few patients accepted further treatment. To solve this problem, I studied sales. Initially I didn't like the idea of the dentist being a salesperson. But isn't this the reaction of most professionals when you try to convince them they are salespeople, too? I focused mainly on the works of Tom Hopkins, and after studying for several months I realized that it was not about luring people into buying the wrong things at all, but rather about communicating to them honestly the treatment I was proposing, and why I believed it was best for them.

But I felt the need to become more efficient at educating my patients about their treatment plans. I went on to study communications, reading more books and listening to more tapes. Then one day, I came to understand an interesting concept: I thought that the essence of communication had to be advertising.

To me, scientific advertising seemed to be very similar to scientific management. Advertisers split-run their ads in newspapers and magazines. They check the results, reject the less productive ad, and keep the more productive one, and then this ad will run against a newly created one. They keep perfecting their language and style continuously, just as I hoped to do in communicating with my patients and staff.

I remembered what worked well and what generated the least number of questions. I rejected what proved not to be clear and generated further questions. This technique worked very well for me and I think helped us grow from two chairs to five in just a couple of years. Getting enough patients for the practice was no longer a problem.

People

As a lean leader, I must respect people—their intelligence, time, experience, knowledge, and integrity. It sounds almost too basic to even mention, but is not basic at all. In fact it's proven to be *the most fundamental and challenging part* of our lean transformation. It's very encouraging to me that this is supported by Fujio Cho, the Chairman of Toyota Motor Company. He states that there are just three keys to becoming a lean leader:

- **Go see:** Go to the place where the work is done and value created
- **Ask why:** Look for root causes, not symptoms
- **Show respect:** Respect for people's knowledge, ideas, and time

I believe that the first two items on Chairman Cho's short list are actually just other ways of showing respect for everyone in an organization. I show respect every time I leave my office and go to where the work is actually done—the gemba. Asking those who do the work *why* a problem has occurred or a situation exists is yet another way of showing respect for their knowledge and experience.

Following these three "simple" principles is a tremendous challenge because of the discipline that it takes to follow them every day. However, the payback for adhering to them has been tremendous because it made everyone in the practice a partner in our lean transformation. This takes even more dedication than focusing on purpose and process because engaging people is a daily commitment to a new culture. But ultimately a lean transformation occurs only when this new lean culture becomes a way of life. *How did we achieve this level of engagement and partnership?*

Show Respect for People and Their Personal Lives

In 1985, one of Mahatma Gandhi's ideas attracted me. He believed that every decision that does not show respect for the people it affects is necessarily wrong. One day I was sitting in my office at Antonine University in Beirut with a professor. He was a close friend and we talked openly. A secretary came into the office with a letter containing a decision from upper management that I would need to implement. I don't recall exactly what it was. I remember, however, that I had discussed the wishes of the teachers, employees, and students with the dean prior to him making his decision. For some unknown reason, he had not taken any of their proposals into consideration. As a result, now I was expected to ask people to behave in a way that did not fit their beliefs. "I need to go talk to the dean," I told my friend. "This decision lacks respect for our people." Clearly, I had adopted Gandhi's idea as a guiding post.

Gandhi's idea seems rooted in a culture of respect for life in general. It reflects his personal philosophy and beliefs. I realize now that this principle was instilled in me at a very early age. The middle and high schools I attended in Beirut were run by Marist French monks. They promoted respect for every human being and treated us as their equals. In middle school, I remember being asked to serve on a committee of a dozen students who helped the principal run the school. We represented the "voice of the students." Brother Francois, the principal, wanted to learn about everything the students needed and did everything he could to improve life at the school. Tolerance for diversity and acceptance of others' opinions were some of the Marist school's moral values and Brother Francois and the other monks led by example.

I mention this because lean leaders are increasingly vocal today about the necessity of "respect for people." This idea is fundamental to the Toyota way. In my opinion, Toyota's interpretation of this idea cannot be fully understood without considering Toyota's culture. When I read what different authors and lean leaders think about the concept, they always have slightly different interpretations.

In fact, the interpretation of the "respect for people" principle is subject to every person's set of values—personal, social, religious, ethical, etc. Because I have never been exposed to the "respect for people" at Toyota, I can only attempt to describe how we do it at Bahri Dental Group, hoping that our philosophy is similar to Toyota's. I find it helpful to use the metaphor of a garden. After the gardener decides which plants and flowers should be planted, his job becomes to water every plant and give each one the nutrients it needs to flourish. He might predict that an apple tree will give him apples, and naturally he expects that the quality of those apples will change from season to season because of a variety of environmental conditions.

At our office we try to create an environment for our employees to prosper and flourish. Their performance on the job varies somewhat over time as a result of outside conditions. No matter how hard they try to keep their personal problems outside the office, I have found that is nearly impossible. Instead of blaming them for bringing personal problems to work, we try to respect that these things happen and occasionally help each other solve them. Interdependence is one of our guiding principles. Simply recognizing that I need my staff as much as they need me has been a good step toward dealing with employees as true partners in the business.

The respect concept was reinforced in a discussion with my older brother, George, an orthopedic surgeon with a big heart and a lot of wisdom when it comes to human relations. I was complaining to him about my assistants using the phone for personal calls more than I would like them to. I was thinking about asking them to limit those calls to lunch time so they won't disturb the schedule. "Don't they have families?" he said. "You can't stop people from worrying about their families just because they work for you."

This helped me understand that my business could not provide for my family without providing for my employees' families first. I started making my decisions starting from that concept, and I learned it better by practice. Their babies, spouses, parents, and siblings are all part of our collective lives. Whenever they need to help any of them, the whole team comes together to fill in for their teammates and allow them to care for their loved ones.

This is reinforced in Stephen Covey's *The 7 Habits of Highly Effective People*, in which he describes the evolution of relationships between staff and management, from dependence to independence to interdependence. Interdependence happens when two independent people, who can very well be successful separately, voluntarily join efforts and become even more successful together. In other words, when it comes to my employees, they are my customers and I am theirs. My goal is to make their life in my office better than in any other office so I won't lose them to the competition. I encourage them to think the same way, to ensure that they are the best people for our business needs. I believe they are essentially contracting professionals who choose to be with us because we are their best option at this time. In the end, it's a relationship based on mutual respect and need.

Create an Open Business Partnership

Our goal is to create a long-term partnership with our employees. Long-term employment is a blessing because it reduces the necessity for training new employees and keeps the environment stable and the staff cohesive, but it also creates challenges for the business. For example, even if the office's productivity is not continuously improving, employees still expect a salary increase every year. Unless the business is growing dramatically each year, this is a big challenge.

When I felt this problem creeping up on us, I chose to discuss it openly with my staff. I started the meeting by saying, "At your yearly review this year, if you intend not to ask for a salary raise, please raise your hand." Obviously no hands were raised. "Every year," I continued, "the raises you ask for together equal the salaries of one to two full-time employees. We have dealt with it so far by not replacing the employees who have left the office. If we keep following the same policy, no employees will be left here. If we are to afford keeping you for a long time, our only option is to find ways to make everyone more productive."

In this meeting I was dealing with staff as partners in the business, recognizing that we all want better lives for our families. Since that moment, we are more focused on reducing waste and increasing productivity, so I could afford giving them raises when they are due.

I used to hate the fact that when a patient canceled you have nothing to do and then you'd get bored and then you don't feel like working for the rest of the day. But here, there's always something you can do.

— Kelly Sundberg
Dental Hygienist

To reach our goals, I have to be open to their ideas, and they have to be open to mine. We simply have to bring to the surface the problems that hinder productivity and work together on eliminating them.

When did we decide to place "respect for people" at the center of our management system? I can't really tell, but going back through some of our meeting briefings, I found an interesting quote by our very first front desk assistant. She had planned our monthly meetings schedule for 1991, less than a year after the practice was started. At the end of a list of dates for each meeting she wrote: *Please come to the meetings prepared to share ideas. This office is always open to discuss ideas for improvement.* Reading her remarks 17 years later made me feel confident about the deep roots of our respect for employees and their ideas.

Respect *Everyone's* Time

Showing respect for our patients' busy schedule is normal; our livelihood depends on their satisfaction. We spent years developing a system in which they won't have to wait for us. But should employees wait? If we think about respect for people, we need to think about *all* people. That's why we extended the no-wait policy to staff as well. In dentistry, one of the most frequent complaints comes from hygienists having to wait for dentists to check their patients' teeth. In one of our meetings we discussed the staff-waiting problem. It is a simple fact that our lives are made out of time. Making people wait would be like stealing an irreplaceable part of their life. We then created a simple slogan to extend the respect for people's time concept to the staff also: *People shouldn't have to wait.*

The hygienist, the patient, the assistant, the dentist, the front desk assistant, the lab technician … they're all people and they shouldn't have to wait. When our lean practitioner friends visit the office, they often see the most visible part of the system, the very short patient-waiting time. Although not as visible to visitors, the staff non-waiting time is equally as important and it came as a result of our synchronization efforts.

Eliminating unnecessary steps to reduce the workers' burden was most efficiently achieved after we understood the just-in-time (JIT) and overproduction concepts. JIT requires that we exert only the required efforts at the moment they are needed. Overproduction represents any effort defying the JIT definition. It follows that fighting overproduction would be a great way to reduce human efforts so that employees would believe that lean is really there to make their lives easier, not harder.

An example to illustrate this point is a kaizen project the front desk assistants worked on. The insurance coordinator was confirming insurance eligibility and remaining benefits for each patient. She would verify today's patients, then tomorrow's, then the day after that, etc., until the end of the month. When she reached that point, the schedule would have changed so much that she would have to go back to verify insurance eligibility and remaining benefits again for today's patient, tomorrow's patients, and so on.

Verifying insurance was her full-time job. In the kaizen project, she studied the time it takes to verify the benefits with each insurance company. Some companies had lists we could access with our computer system; their clients could be verified in 30 seconds or less.

At the other extreme, some insurance companies required a phone call and could take up to 30 minutes to verify the information. She classified the insurance companies into four categories according to the time it took to verify the patient information with them. The less-than-30-seconds and the less-than-five-minutes categories did not need to be verified before the patient arrived to the office. The others would be verified one day before the appointment. We call this JIT insurance verification.

One day she came to my office and said, "Look at this, Dr Bahri! I have calculated the time it took me to verify insurance … three and a half hours."

"Great!" I said, "You have cut your day in half."

"No," she answered, "That's three and half hours *a month*."

This shows you the impact of just one project aimed at reducing human efforts.

Gain Trust by Providing Proof
My dad's brother, George, Sr., was a man of character. He was honest, outspoken, and never compromised his principles. Every son in our family saw him as a role model for strength, decisiveness, and clarity of thought. Once he had an opinion he expressed it very clearly and defended it for as long as he needed to. In many instances in which I needed courage in my life, I remembered him and thought of what he would do in that particular situation. I considered him stubborn and being stubborn seemed to work for him, so I thought it should work for me as well.

Then everything changed the day he became ill with a very aggressive cancer. The doctor said that he most likely had three months to live, and he turned out to be right. My giant, powerful uncle crumbled very quickly to become a weak little body. He lived his last days in horrible pain. But in spirit he remained the same noble, honest, out-spoken man.

By this time most of his family had left Lebanon because of the civil war, so I decided to take on fewer patients and take care of him, along with his wife and children, while he was ill. During one of our quiet chats, he told me some of his life stories and emphasized how flexible and open-minded he was. I couldn't stop myself from laughing.

"You laugh because you think I'm stubborn," he said. "Convince me of your idea, and you'll see that I will defend it as fiercely as I was defending mine!"

Little did he know that he changed my life with those words. I realized then that no one will continue to be stubborn if you can effectively prove to them your point of view. Proof is what is needed to change people's behavior. From that moment with my uncle I have never asked anyone to trust me simply because I believe I know better. I have always tried to work together with people to find out whether our ideas are valid or not.

Build Consensus Rather Than Attempt to Control

I have no doubt in my mind that my experience at the dental school is the richest in my life, that it literally molded me into the person I am today. If I was able to implement lean thinking in my office, it is clearly because I had helped implement many projects at the school during my 10 years there. I surely had less experience back then, but I was exposed to wonderful people with extraordinary talents in dentistry and management, as well as in human relationships.

Authority was a loose term back then, with the government rendered incapacitated due to the deep divisions among the different sections of the Lebanese population. My position gave me formal authority that I could use as I liked in my daily operations until it conflicted with the interest of some political party member. In this case, pressure would start to build up against me and animosity could grow fast. I had to use my authority very judicially, keeping an appearance of strength and clarity, but deep down I knew that any *faux pas* on my part could become dangerous.

What was the solution? Consensus. To build consensus I had to discuss every matter with the people it affected. Failure to do so would, at minimal, bring me a lot of headaches. It took me a little while to understand the formula, but once I did, managing became much easier. I was nevertheless tired of having to consult with every person before I could make a decision. Another factor bothered me enormously. Because we all were government employees, once staff members were hired, there was almost no way to fire them. If people weren't doing their jobs properly, I had to find ways to convince them to change their behavior.

When I came to live in the United States in 1990, my first desire was to use my freedom to make decisions without fear, and this meant firing whoever did not perform well on the job. To me, this was real freedom, real authority. I was quick to find out though that using authority just because I was the one signing the checks did not lead to a prospering business. Firing people because they did not follow my command only led me to have to hire new employees who ended up behaving like the people I just fired. The only difference was I had to train the new employees all over again.

Using my authority during the early days at my Jacksonville office was leading me nowhere; therefore, I decided that the way I lived with my employees in Lebanon was more appropriate. I went back to building consensus and motivating people to do their jobs rather than using command-and-control. I took genuine interest in my staff's interests and decided that our business should improve my employees' lives as much as it did my own.

Decide to Become a Leader

With all the literature on leadership, I have always wondered what personality type is best-suited for success as a leader. Media told me it had a lot to do with personal charisma. Political leaders, for example, often have outstanding oratory skills. This is what I thought leadership meant.

I always wondered how those leaders ran their private lives. What were they like when away from the public eye? *Management of the Absurd* by Richard Farson looked at the matter from an interesting angle. Farson submits that any personality can succeed and looking for particular traits is really a waste of time.

Essentially he tells us to stop wasting time on personality analysis and just go do what needs to be done. This concept is reinforced by a quote I have always attributed to Goethe, "Whatever you can do, or dream you can do, begin it. Boldness has genius, power, and magic in it!" It is action-oriented and inspires me to create, change, and improve. It is like the Nike "Just do it" slogan.

Experimenting with new management systems like lean, Total Quality Management, and process reengineering was an adventure. I felt like a little boy following a bird in a jungle. As I went deeper, I became more fascinated by the beauty I discovered around me. But I also feared the unknown. *What if I went too far to find at the end that I was ruining my business? Would my patients accept my new methods? Would my employees agree to all of the changes along the way?*

This kind of questioning has the potential to become paralyzing at times. Whenever I've felt doubt, the answer was there: *Just do it.*

Conclusion

I am including here a handful of lessons I've learned in the hopes of keeping your lean efforts focused. These lessons have worked well for us and I welcome you to use them, but please also improve upon them and create your own.

- Improve the process flow before you eliminate waste from individual operations. Start improvements close to the customer and spread the improvements backward toward the beginning of the value stream. Some operations can be totally eliminated, meaning you may never have to work on them.

- Run your value-adding operations in a series and the support functions in parallel. While your value-added operations (e.g., crown or filling in our case) are running, your support functions (e.g., writing notes in the chart) can happen in parallel.

- Start small when making improvements within your organization. This way any mistakes you make will have only minor impact. Change is also most effective when it grows naturally like a human embryo. Like the embryo, change needs to start small, drawing upon as few resources as possible, before it can expand outward to encompass the entire organization. Often we tend to start on a large scale because we think in batch-and-queue terms, even when implementing change.

- Use these small-scale experiments to prove to your coworkers that the changes you are proposing are actually improvements. Providing proof changes minds, establishes trust, and reduces any resistance to change.

- Look for flexibility in your processes so you can respond faster to market changes. Look for flexibility in your people—flexibility to learn and to help whenever and wherever they are needed. This is the best way to constantly increase your organization's capacity.

- Put the decision makers together rather than in separate locations. Communication and decision-making will improve dramatically.

Most importantly, *learn*. However you can, learn. I have found that learning is even more fun than teaching. When I was in college, my friends and I continuously shared new knowledge with each other. When I began learning lean management, I explored new knowledge first with an interested individual and then with everyone on the staff. Today, I'm always adding to my network of fellow lean learners from around the world, so that I can learn more and more creative lean applications. My only plan is to keep learning. My wish is that every leader becomes a lifelong lean learner and teacher.

But start implementing lean today. Do not wait until you have learned "all about lean," including the leadership principles I've written about here. In the end, practice is the only thing that will enable you to *find* your own way by *learning* your own way. These personal lessons will determine the kind of leader that you will become.

Acknowledgments

"Lean dentistry" and this book grew by the efforts of everyone who worked at Bahri Dental Group over the past 19 years. I learned from everyone. From those who had their doubts, I learned flexibility; from those who have been flexible enough to give lean a try, the power of learning together. Some have seen the dream come true, and others have left to pursue different dreams.

Jerry Bussell, thank you! You discovered our lean practice and in a very generous effort called Jim Womack, John Shook, and many others and introduced us to them. You also introduced me to Michael Brassard—and the project for this book was born. I will always value your friendship and your selflessness. You are a true lean leader!

Dr. Michael Dagher, MD, introduced me to TQM. Michael, thank you for triggering the long learning experience that led me to finding lean dentistry.

Big thanks to my brother and partner, Dr. Gaby Bahri, for listening to my same lean stories, year after year.

Special thanks to my brother-in-law, Dr. Robert Helt, DDS. From Paris you shared your management experience, your ideas, and your French wine. They were all invaluable.

My dear friend, Dr. B.J. Barakat, MD, you listened to my ideas and gave me yours. I value your friendship and your thinking.

I thank Jim Womack for believing in our work and helping us spread the word about it.

John Shook, thank you for your support and encouragement.

Dave LaHote and Chet Marchwinski, for helping us and the lean community better understand the improvements we have made by your thoughtful questions and careful documentation of our work.

My editor, Alexis Schroeder, worked relentlessly, always with an uplifting attitude—and never laughing at my writing in my presence. She guided me through the steps of creating this book with incredible patience and grace. Thank you, Lex, for all your time and work.

Working with Michael Brassard is a true privilege. I am lucky to have found a critic with your exquisite thinking precision and your elegant style. Thank you.

My gratitude and respect go to my parents, Abdo and Chafica Bahri. My love goes to Salime, Amal, Georges, Nabil, Fady, Gaby, Nawal, Liliane, Andre, and their families.

My love and respect to my in-laws, Rachid and Siham Baz, and to Nicole and Paula and their families.

About the Author

Dr. Sami Bahri, DDS, runs a Jacksonville, FL, private dental practice that includes three general dentists, one orthodontist, 10 chairs for general dentistry, and seven chairs for orthodontics.

His desire to know how other industries manage resources to deliver value to customers led him to study Total Quality Management, Six Sigma, and ultimately, in 1996, lean management after reading *Lean Thinking* by James Womack and Daniel Jones. By 2006, Bahri Dental Group provided the same amount of dental treatments as 2005, but needed 40% less resources, thanks to the application of "lean dental management." In 2007, he presented his work as a keynote speaker at the Shingo Prize Conference where he was recognized as the "World's First Lean Dentist." He lectures nationally and internationally on implementing lean management in dentistry.

Dr. Bahri was born in Lebanon where he received his dental degree from the Saint Joseph Jesuit Dental School in 1977. He then spent three years at the University of Paris, specializing in dental prosthodontics. After returning to Lebanon, he opened his first dental practice, began teaching dentistry, and in 1984 became the founding director of a new dental school at the Lebanese University. In 1990, Dr Bahri moved to Jacksonville where he launched his practice.

Bibliography

Berry, Leonard L. and A. Parasuraman. *Marketing Services: Competing Through Quality*. New York: Free Press, 1991.

Blanchard, Kenneth H. and Spencer Johnson. *The One Minute Manager*. New York: William Morrow & Company, 1981.

Covey, Stephen R. *The 7 Habits of Highly Effective People*. New York: Free Press, 1990.

Crosby, Philip B. *Quality is Free*. New York: Signet, 1980.

Csíkszentmihályi, Mihály. *Flow: The Psychology of Optimal Experience*. New York: HarperCollins, 1990.

Deming, W. Edwards. *Out of the Crisis*. Cambridge, MA: MIT Press, 1982.

Drucker, Peter. *The Effective Executive*. New York: Harper & Row, 1967.

Farson, Richard. *Management of the Absurd*. New York: Free Press, 1997.

Gerber, Michael. *The E-Myth: Why Most Small Businesses Don't Work and What To Do About It*. New York: Harper Business, 1988.

Hammer, Michael. *Reengineering the Corporation: A Manifesto for Business Revolution*. New York: HarperCollins, 1993.

Hammer, Michael. *Reengineering Management: The Mandate for New Leadership*. New York: HarperCollins, 1995.

Harris, Rick, Chris Harris, and Earl Wilson. *Making Materials Flow*. Cambridge, MA: Lean Enterprise Institute, 2003.

Hopkins, Tom. *How to Master the Art of Selling*. New York: Warner Books, 1982.

Hopkins, Tom. *Low Profile Selling*. Scottsdale, AZ: Tom Hopkins International, 1994.

Imai, Masaaki. *Kaizen: The Key to Japan's Competitive Success*. New York: McGraw-Hill, 1986.

Japan Management Association. *Kanban Just-In-Time at Toyota: Management Begins at the Workplace*. New York: Productivity Press, 1986.

LeBoeuf, Michael. *Getting Results: The Secret to Motivating Yourself and Others*. New York: Berkeley Publishing Group, 1986.

LeBoeuf, Michael. *How to Win Customers and Keep Them for Life*. New York: Berkeley Books, 1987.

Liker, Jeffrey. *The Toyota Way*. New York: McGraw-Hill, 2004.

Ohno, Taiichi. *The Toyota Production System: Beyond Large-Scale Production*. New York: Productivity Press, 1988.

Peters, Thomas J. and Robert H. Waterman. *In Search of Excellence: Lessons from America's Best-Run Companies*. New York: Warner Books, 1984.

Rother, Mike and Rick Harris. *Creating Continuous Flow*. Cambridge, MA: Lean Enterprise Institute, 2001.

Rother, Mike and John Shook. *Learning to See*. Cambridge, MA: Lean Enterprise Institute, 2003.

Shingo, Shigeo. *A Study of the Toyota Production System: From an Engineering Viewpoint*. New York: Productivity Press, 1989.

Senge, Peter. *The Fifth Discipline: The Art and Practice of the Learning Organization*. New York: Broadway Business, 2006.

Sewell, Carl and Paul B. Brown. *Customers for Life: How to Turn That One-Time Buyer Into a Lifetime Customer*. New York: Pocket Books, 1990.

Smalley, Art. *Creating Level Pull*. Cambridge, MA: Lean Enterprise Institute, 2004.

Treacy, Michael and Fred Wiersema. *The Discipline of Market Leaders: Choose Your Customers, Narrow Your Focus, Dominate Your Market*. New York: Perseus Books, 1995.

Walton, Mary. *The Deming Management Method*. New York: Putnam, 1986.

Walton, Sam. *Made in America*, New York: Bantam Books, 1993.

Womack, James P. and Daniel T. Jones. *Lean Thinking*. New York: Simon & Schuster, 1996.

Womack, James P. and Daniel T. Jones. *The Machine that Changed the World*. New York: Scribner, 1990.

Womack, James P. and Daniel T. Jones. *Seeing the Whole*. Cambridge, MA: Lean Enterprise Institute, 2002.

The Lean Lexicon, 4th Edition: A Graphical Glossary for Lean Thinkers. Edited by Chet Marchwinski and Alexis Schroeder. Cambridge, MA: Lean Enterprise Institute, 2008.